A Double Dose of Dilaudid
Real Stories from a Small-Town ER

Kerry Hamm

Copyright © 2015
All Rights Reserved.

Disclaimer:
Names, locations, and portions of the details included in this book have been altered to protect the privacy of those involved.

Edited for quality purposes after publication

Welcome to a small-town Emergency Room in Ohio. With six trauma bays, one mental health room, one low pressure room, one quarantine room, and 11 other exam bays, this ER has the capacity to fit 21 patients at a time, with more than 100 patients often lining up in the lobby and waiting room on any given evening shift.

We're no big-shot inner city hospital. We transfer out burns and severe pediatric cases. We have a mental health floor, inpatient rehab, intermediate care/critical care, and hospice floor in addition to pediatrics, general surgery, obstetrics, and nursery floors. Unless patients are directly admitted from facilities in surrounding areas, they show up in our department first. Typically, we don't see many gunshot wounds or stabbings, but what does come through the doors keeps us all on our toes.

My name is Kerry and I'm the first person you'll see when you come through those ER doors: registration. Two to three clerks work during the day and evening shifts, taking turns gathering names, birth dates, and diagnoses at the front (while juggling floor transfers, admits from surrounding hospitals, and outside phone calls from some cat lady named Linda who's making her third call this shift to see if we think she needs to come in for tingling in her left butt cheek), and then in the back, where we enter patients' rooms to gather contact and insurance information to complete the registration process. Once 11 p.m. hits, I wave to my coworkers as they walk out the door, and I'm left at the registration desk with a triage nurse in a small room behind the desk, security lurking behind a two-way mirror that takes up an entire wall in front of the registration desk, a not-so-empty waiting room to my right, and six registered nurses and one or two doctors in the back.

Every story here is true, though dialogue has been changed slightly, all names have been changed, and some situations have been slightly altered to protect patient privacy.

Cheat Sheet

Readers have brought to my attention that some of the terms I use in my books are confusing, meaning my readers can't fully enjoy the stories. I plan to edit my previous editions to include this 'cheat sheet' of terms I frequently use.

MVA: Motor Vehicle Accident

ETOH: ethyl alcohol is the real meaning of this, but in our ER this means our patient is drunk

CC/cc: chief complaint

Tones dropping: a series of melodic beeps play before dispatch alerts medics of a patient's call. Most of us groan when we hear the tones because we know we're getting another patient.

Stemi: a procedure in which a patient is

taken to the Cath Lab to clear a cardiac blockage. From what I understand, this is done by making an incision near the groin rather than entering through the heart itself.

Face sheet/facesheet: a piece of paper detailing the patient's name, contact information, next of kin, primary physician, chief complaint, and insurance information. One copy must go to the back, the other to our tray. Then, another must go to medics, the floor (if a patient is admitted), and the coroner (if it comes down to that).

NOK: next of kin

DID: died in department

DOA: dead on arrival

BAC: blood alcohol content

Bus: another term for ambulance

If I have forgotten to include any terms you feel others may not recognize, feel free to leave a review with your suggestion!

Prancing in the Pumpkin Patch

There were four days left until Halloween night, and the mid-Ohio weather had chilled substantially in comparison to the 70-degrees we were feeling the week before. Patients presenting injuries sustained outside waned off considerably with the dropping temperatures. To be honest, I couldn't recall coming across such an injury all week, and staff members welcomed the change, fully knowing we would be slammed from floor to ceiling with patients once ice and snow came along just a few weeks later. With an hour left on the last shift of my week-long stretch, I headed to the back and grabbed my cart. The tracking board was not overloaded, but there were enough rooms to keep me busy for a good half hour. I was tired and sore; the last thing I wanted to do was walk from room to room, exposing myself to all of the cold and cough diagnoses that seemed to be the chief complaint of nearly all the patients I needed to see.

I scanned the board for the nearest room but my attention darted back to the center of the board. The diagnosis was a simple one: injury to left ankle. Never one to shy away from an injury, I dragged my cart over to the patient's room. The 30-something-year-old female had been placed in a room reserved for less urgent traumas.

"Registration," I announced when I knocked on the door.

"You can come in."

She sounded nice and free of pain.

Her room's overhead lights were turned off and she was sitting upright in her bed. As I moved further into the room, the patient used her remote to mute the television that was suspended in the upper left corner. She smoothed over her thick, wiry brown hair with the palm of her right hand before scratching at the tip of her nose. Her almond eyes were tired and her eyelids heavy. She pushed the fleece-lined sleeves of her gray sweatshirt to her pointy elbows.

"So, did I break it?" she asked with a brittle chuckle. She nodded to her left ankle. The left leg of the patient's jeans was rolled up in a bulge to her knee, exposing her smooth, milky leg and swollen, red joint.

I shrugged, "Sorry, but they don't really tell me much. I'm mostly in charge of making sure your address and insurance information is accurate so your bill doesn't get sent to your house."

She nodded in understanding. "Bet you're wondering what I did, huh?"

Of course I was. She was reading my mind.

I glanced to her ankle and ran through a few scenarios: the patient tripped as she was going down the stairs; she was walking her dog and it took off, wrapping its leash around her ankle; she was playing softball with work colleagues and stepped down the wrong way. There were dozens of ways she could have injured herself. But I wasn't quite prepared to what *really* happened.

"Well," I said, "we do have to go over an accident screen. Do you want to do that part first?"

The patient nodded.

I clicked and clacked at my keyboard and mouse until I reached the accident screen page.

"Okay," I chirped. "Did this happen at work?"

"Nope. Pumpkin patch."

I nodded. "Okay. And what happened? Did you just trip?"

The patient began laughing hysterically, embarrassed by what she was about to tell me. She grabbed at her stomach.

"Oh," she said with a grin. "I think that counts as a workout."

I smiled and hoped her story was as good as she thought it was.

"Well," she said, "I have nine kids."

"Nine kids?" I exclaimed. "Wow, you must have such a busy life."

Now, I wasn't judging the patient, but I sure was trying to do the math in my head.

"Two sets of twins and the newest one is six months' tomorrow. And my husband decided he wanted to go sow some oats with his girlfriend, so he moved out and I've been doing the best I can."

I nodded. "Wow."

"Yeah, and with Halloween coming up. Well, you know...Pumpkins are expensive. I mean, how is it fair that the good pumpkins are, like, six bucks a piece? If every kid got a pumpkin and then I got one, I'm looking at sixty dollars, at least, just for the pumpkins. I'm a single mom. I work sixty hours a week and most of my pay is taken out in taxes. I was just trying to give my kids the best Halloween."

I knew to keep my mouth shut. She was having a moment and was afraid of being judged. Little did she know; I didn't care about the rest. I just wanted to know what really happened.

"My mom said she'd watch the kids tonight," she explained, "and my sister said she'd go with me. So we went out to the pumpkin patch after dark—you know, it's that one right off the highway outside of town."

I didn't know, but I nodded anyway.

"I figured, 'Who's gonna miss a few pumpkins?'"

She looked to me for a response when she asked, "Well, am I right?"

My eyes widened and I nodded nervously, but

I hid my unease with a bright smile. "Well, yeah. I mean, nobody would probably even notice, right? It's not like you were hurting anyone."

"Exactly," she said loudly, relieved to hear someone agreed with her.

"Well," she continued, "We were walking around, right, looking for pumpkins. But then we saw a cop car."

"Uh-oh."

She rolled her eyes. "Yeah. When we saw it, we tried to run. What am I supposed to do if I get arrested?"

It was a rhetorical question.

"Okay," she said with a smile. "So this car turned towards us and I did the only thing I knew to do: I ran. Well," she hesitated, "I tried to run."

She pointed to her ankle. "And that's when my foot got caught on a vine."

The patient smacked her palms together. "BAM! I went down."

"Did the cop stop?" I asked.

She laughed so hard her cheeks turned red and she wheezed.

"No," she replied. "Turns out it wasn't even a cop. It was someone else there to do the same thing I was doing."

The patient left with a badly-sprained ankle and a cushioned boot. We estimated the cost of her visit at close to three thousand dollars.

Natural Selection

About a week after the pumpkin patch incident, I was in the back, trying to catch up on the overwhelming number of patients visiting the Emergency Room. Every room I tried to enter had a doctor or nurse inside except for one with a diagnosis of: attacked by a skunk.

Now, I had seen other strange animal diagnoses: attacked by a chicken (still, to this day, I recall playing Zelda games on my Nintendo GameBoy, swinging Link's sword at a few chickens until they became overly-frustrated and finally pecked away one of my lives); charged by a cow; and one of my favorites: knocked down by a puppy. I had never, though, had the opportunity to speak to anyone attacked by a skunk. I wondered what the patient's definition of 'attack' was, and then I raised my nose to the air and sniffed, trying to pick up on stinky scent as I wheeled my cart to the nurse's station directly outside the patient's door.

"Did they say how it happened?" I questioned the unit clerk.

She was thumbing through a lopsided pile of paperwork and shook her head.

"I don't smell it," I noted. "Did it spray him?"

She shook her head again. "Nope. I guess it

just bit him."

"Was it a pet?"

"Nope."

"Well," I said sarcastically, "it's not like skunks give us a sign to stay away from them, like *spraying*."

The unit clerk laughed. "Well, let me know what happened when you find out. We've been taking bets on what the guy was doing."

I knocked on the door and was welcomed to enter.

The patient was a 40-something-year-old male. His once-white tee shirt, now stained by splotches of old mustard and oil, was drenched in smelly sweat. The man's wide forehead was glossy and his skin was beet red. His breathing was shallow and rapid, and with each breath his large stomach jiggled.

"Hi," I said. "I'm here from registration."

"Am I going to die from this?" he worriedly questioned.

I bit my lower lip and felt my eyebrows and forehead scrunch. I wanted to mess with him and say grimly, "I'm afraid it doesn't look good."

But I didn't.

"I think there would be a few more doctors and nurses in here if they thought you were going to die," I truthfully responded.

He held up his left hand and showed me the bite mark. There were several pink puncture wounds to the flesh between his sausage thumb and index finger. The area was so red it appeared to be burned, and puss was already oozing from the man's wounds.

"Look what the thing did," he ordered angrily.

"How did this happen?" I asked cautiously.

The man took a deep breath, which was followed by a series of whooping coughs.

"See," he said, "I was walking behind Wal Mart."

"Like, just to walk?" I interrupted. "Or were you looking for something?"

He shook his head. "I was just walking off steam. My truck broke down. I think it's the damn fuel pump. But, anyway, I was waiting for the tow truck to come. I saw this skunk hanging out by the dumpster, right, so I called to it."

The man mimicked his calls to the wild animal by smooching his lips and clicking his tongue.

"Did it come to you?"

He nodded. "Yep. The thing just walked right up to me."

The patient's claim concerned me, especially because our location was considered to be rural. Most people in the area possess common knowledge regarding wildlife. For example, most small animals in the area usually shy away from humans, unless they are conditioned to human presence via feeding or the most alarming concern: the animals have rabies. Judging by the patient's story, he was not concerned when the animal approached him.

"And then it attacked you? Was it a baby?" I asked.

He shook his head. "Nope. I leaned down and it let me pick it up. Wasn't a baby, either. It was the size of my wife's cat, I think it was."

My mouth fell open in awe. "You picked up a wild skunk?"

And then he looked at me like *I* was stupid. "Well, *yeah*. It came right to me."

"And then it bit you," I said dryly. I had meant to ask a question, but it simply didn't happen that way.

"Not right away," he gently argued. "See, I was petting its head and stroking it around the ears. So then I tried to pet its back and..."

The man whipped his head to the left and chomped at the air.

"It took a good chunk from my hand. I'm telling you," he said, "that I threw that thing so hard it's probably over in Illinois right now."

I moved to nod.

"And now," said the patient, "I'm going to die. I'm going to die and everyone's going to remember me as the guy who got killed from a skunk bite."

He was becoming panicky and loud. The man squirmed in bed and retched.

"This stuff they gave me isn't working. I think they gave me something like thirteen shots. And none of it's working. You gotta tell someone that I'm dying. You'll get someone for me, right?"

"As soon as we get through your chart," I promised, "I'll ask your nurse to come see you. Would that be okay?"

The man agreed.

In the end, the patient received 16 shots. The good news? He didn't die, and as he was waiting in the lobby for his wife to come pick him up, he swore he'd never attempt to pick up another skunk again.

Penis Problem

Near the end of one of my overnight shifts, a man walked through the front door and approached the counter. There was a deep level of pain expressed on his 40-year-old face, but I couldn't tell what was ailing the man. He didn't nurse either arm or favor a certain leg. He didn't clutch at his sides or place his hand over his heart.

"I need to see a doctor," he announced in a broken voice.

I took the man's name and date of birth.

"Do you have a primary physician?" I asked.

He shook his head and I noticed a bead of sweat roll down his smooth forehead. His eyes were clear and he didn't reek of alcohol, so I figured he wasn't drunk or high.

"And what seems to be the problem this morning?"

The man hesitated. "I'd rather not say."

"Sir," I assured the patient, "anything you say will not be judged or repeated. But I have to put something in the diagnosis screen so our charge nurse can assign the proper room for your needs."

He looked away and repeated, "I'd just rather not say. I don't want anyone to laugh."

I prepared myself for the typical diagnoses of

someone who utters those words. Usually, the patient at the desk shies away and finally mentions something like 'pain during urination' or something equally embarrassing to the patient but nothing I haven't heard before.

"We're here to help you," I calmly stated. "None of our staff members will laugh at you. And," I encouraged him, "we've heard it all. There's nothing you can say to me that someone else hasn't told me."

His toffee eyes met mine for but a moment. The man then looked to the tile floor.

"My, uh," he whispered. "My penis hurts."

I nodded. "Okay. Now, if you can just sign the top line of our consent form so we can treat you, a nurse should be up for you in just a moment."

The man signed the consent form and I signed as a witness. Before I even placed a label on the form, a nurse had appeared from the back. She was patiently waiting to lead the man to a room.

"I don't want people to laugh at me," he said to her.

The head nurse on duty that night was and still is the kindest, most professional nurse I've ever met. She didn't break the slightest smile, but instead shook her head and told the man, "Absolutely not. We're here to help."

I made a copy of the man's consent form.

Before I could sit down again, he and the head nurse disappeared to the back. I sat down and greeted hospital employees arriving for the start of their six a.m. shifts.

The phone rang.

I immediately recognized the number as coming from the charge nurse's phone.

"Whatcha need?" I asked, believing I had forgotten something or had made a mistake.

"I need you to stop what you're doing and come back here to get that last patient's information," she said hurriedly. "He's going to surgery as soon as you're done."

"But it hasn't even been five minutes," I noted aloud.

"I know, but it's serious. I'll send someone up to watch the desk so you can come back here. I really need you to see if he has an emergency contact."

I replied, "Okay, I'll come back right now."

In all the time I worked at the hospital, the quickest discharge happened 20 minutes after the patient arrived. The closest urgency to gather information aside from this patient came from a heart patient coding on the way to the hospital—and even then, family members were waiting in the lobby to give the patient's information. To say I was surprised at the urgency with this patient would be an understatement. I was purely flabbergasted.

When I arrived in the back, most of the nurses were huddled at the center island. Some were giggling. All were whispering.

"What is going on right now?" I asked as I broke the circle.

The head nurse addressed me. "The patient is going to emergency surgery as soon as you're finished getting his information."

"For penis pain?" I questioned in disbelief.

"He's got something stuck in it," another nurse commented.

I needed a second.

"Stuck in it?" I cringed.

The nurse nodded. "He shoved a pen cap up there. Now it's stuck and it's creating problems."

I was still trying to catch my breath.

"He...The man has a *pen cap* stuck in his penis? How...? Why...?"

I cocked my head. "You're kidding me, right?"

The head nurse shook her head and directed me to the patient's room. "No, we're not kidding you. Stuck it in there with the pointy side down."

"But even the top of a pen cap is sharp," I cringed.

The nurse nodded. "I need you to see if he has an emergency contact. Tell me as soon as you're finished, and then we'll get him moved to surgery."

As soon as I entered the patient's room, I wiped the expression of puzzlement from my face.

Tending to business as usual, I gathered information from the patient and acted as if I didn't have a clue to as why he was in the Emergency Room.

"And would you like to add a next of kin or an emergency contact?" I asked.

The man flailed about in his bed, so much that his blue and white hospital gown twisted around his bare legs.

"Nobody can know about this."

The man pointed his finger at me menacingly.

"Nobody can know about this, do you hear me?"

My glance darted from one side of the room to the other. "Uh," I replied nervously, "okay. I can't notify anyone without your permission, sir."

He relaxed. "I'm sorry. Look, I'm sorry for yelling at you. It's just...If my girlfriend finds out that I'm here...and if she finds out *why* I'm here, she's going to kick me out."

The patient pointed over to a chair on the far side of the room. His jeans and tee shirt were both neatly folded atop the furniture.

"My keys are in my pocket," he told me. "Can you maybe move my truck to a different lot so my girlfriend doesn't drive by and see it?"

"Uh, no," I replied. "Sorry, but I can't do that."

"But if she knows it's happened again she's going to make me leave."

I don't know, exactly, what happened to the patient. He was wheeled out of the ER right after I left his room and gave the head nurse a face sheet containing current patient information, and I clocked out of work shortly after speaking with him. I haven't seen the man since. Staff members each had a thought of why the man shoved a pen cap into the tip of his nether-region, but none of us ever knew for sure the patient's reasoning.

Based on a True Story

"Hey, isn't this movie based on a true story?" asked a patient. He pointed to the television. "All of this stuff really happened someplace, right?"

I looked to the television and then back to the patient. I blankly stared at him for a moment, before realizing he was serious.

"Yep," I replied, hiding my amusement. "I do believe it is."

He snapped his fingers and said gloatingly to his wife, "See? I *told* you it really happened."

That movie was *The Green Mile*.

Accidents Happen...

On a somewhat slow evening shift, a mother rushed to the registration desk. She was in tears and was holding an infant in her arms.

"What happened?" my coworker asked before even asking for the patient's name.

The woman motioned to her relaxed child. "We were at home and she fell off the bed. Her head hit the floor so hard that my mom heard it from the kitchen. I don't know how. I was sitting right there. Please, you have to help her."

I glanced up and the baby smiled at me.

Through tears and shouting, the mother gave the child's information to my coworker. Soon, a nurse appeared and walked the mother and child back to an exam room.

"She was really freaking out," I commented to my coworker. "But the baby seemed to be doing okay, yeah?"

"Yeah," he replied. "But I guess it's better to be safe than sorry."

I agreed and went about my business.

Not too long after the patient was registered, I headed to the back to gather information from the child's mother. As usual, I knocked on the door and identified myself. The mother invited me in and I pulled up the patient's chart.

It was instantly clear that the mother was disinterested in registration. She sat at the head of the bed and tapped at the screen of her phone. Her child scooted around the center of the bed. The rails to the bed were down, and I would be lying if I said I wasn't just slightly nervous at the setup.

Each time I asked the patient's mother a question, I had to repeat it twice more.

"Sorry," she laughed. "I'm just trying to keep up with all these Facebook comments."

"It's not a problem," I lied.

I continued with my questions and stared at my screen until the mother would pry her attention away from her phone long enough to finally answer.

As I reached the last question, I found myself feeling excited to leave the room.

"Well," I announced, "I'm finished. So I'm going to make sure the nurses out there get a copy of your paperwo— Oh my God."

The patient's mother didn't even look up. I rushed to the bedside and caught her child in mid-air. In an attempt to explore, the baby crawled to the edge of the bed and was in the process of falling four feet to the hard tile floor.

"Looks like we almost had another accident," I chuckled nervously. I placed the baby back on the bed.

"Oh," said the mother distractedly. "Thanks for catching her. Maybe I should let her crawl around on the floor until it's time to go."

Midnight Madness

It was the second-to-last shift of my workweek and I was grateful that the pace had died down. All week, every shift was unbelievably busy and nearly impossible to keep up with. As the only overnight clerk on duty, I was left with leftover work from previous shifts. Finally, a few minutes after four, I realized all of my work was caught up and I could take a few minutes to myself. No sooner than I filed away my paperwork and sat down, a man walked through the front doors. He held his arms close to his chest, with his hands outstretched. I couldn't help but to be reminded of a t-rex.

"Help," the man groaned.

I stood.

A woman, with her shoelaces untied and dragging under her sneakers, rushed inside and shouted through sobs, "He just jumped out in front of my car. I didn't know what else to do. I swear, he just came out of nowhere and was in front of my car as I was driving."

Believing the man was hit by the woman's vehicle, I moved in closer. When I looked to his hands and scanned over the rest of his badly-bruised and burned body, I knew it was a moment I needed immediate help from the triage nurse.

"Wanda," I called to the back. For the patient's sake, I tried to keep my tone even and my volume just loud enough for the nurse to hear, but when I did not receive an answer, I shouted out more urgently. "Wanda, we really need help out here."

The triage nurse emerged from the exam room located behind the registration desk. As she neared the patient, she saw what I saw: the man had no skin left on his hands or forearms. There was skin missing from his nose and both cheeks, and his shirt was melted to his abdomen. His jeans were singed and the left thigh of his pants had burned, exposing blistered flesh. Any place skin was missing looked like raw packaged chicken breasts from the grocery store. There was no redness to the exposed tendons and muscles. The man moved as little as possible.

"Sit in this chair," the triage nurse directed to the patient.

She positioned a wheelchair just behind him and the man did what he was told without argument.

Instinctively, I pressed the button to the double ER doors to the left of the counter and allowed the nurse entrance to the Emergency Room. I picked up the phone and called to the unit clerk.

"Yeah?" he asked, bored out of his mind. It was clear he hadn't seen the commotion on the cameras that overlooked the lobby and waiting room.

"Wanda's coming back with a trauma. It's pretty bad and she's going to need help. I don't have the patient's name or any information, so you'll have to register him back there. We think he was hit by a car."

The unit clerk and I both hung up.

"Oh no," corrected the panicking woman as she paced the lobby. "I didn't hit him with my car. I was driving and he jumped out in front of me, so I just stopped and brought him in. I don't know him or anything. All I did was help. I swear to God, all I did was help."

"Can you maybe leave your name or the location of where you picked him up?" I asked. "It'd really be helpful."

She pointed to the south end of town. "I just got off the highway. He was just standing there on the exit. Look, I didn't do anything wrong. You can't make me stay, right? I don't want to be responsible for any of this."

It did cross my mind that the woman may have possibly been involved in the matter, but I could not legally hold her hostage, and she was not obligated to provide information about herself or the situation. Once I told her most of that, she bolted, relieved to hear the good news.

As I waited at the desk and stared at the

tracking board for the patient's name to appear, I could hear nurses shouting to one another. I knew better than to call to the back and bother the unit clerk again, and from the direction of the shouts, I could tell the patient had been taken to the decontamination room.

Ten minutes later, the unit clerk came to the front desk.

"Okay," he panted. "He's never been here before, but with a case like this, they told me to bring what I have to you."

Unit Clerks have the ability to register patients and transfer high-risk patients from the ER to another floor, but their registration skills are limited and, although the unit clerks use the same software registration clerks use, they are restricted from certain sections of the program. Because the unit clerk's search for the patient yielded no results for an existing patient file, he and the nurses wanted me to perform an in-depth search. When I did, however, the patient was still showing up as a new patient.

New patients are not incredibly *difficult* to handle, but gathering information from new patients often takes triple the time to fully register than existing patients. While it took virtually no time at all to enter the patient in our system so he could start receiving treatment, I knew it would be next to impossible to gather all the other information I needed, such as contact or insurance information.

I left the patient's chart blank and informed the charge nurse of the situation at hand.

"His girlfriend is on the way," she told me, "and she said she could give you all of his information. Right now, the important thing is that we're able to chart his medications and order lab work."

As I walked from the back to the registration desk, I was careful to stay out of the way of nurses and doctors rushing to and from the patient's room. Every last nurse was involved in treating the newest patient, even when it meant other patients with less serious conditions were left alone for the time being.

Police officers arrived within 10 minutes and walked silently through the lobby and to the back. They questioned the patient while he was still conscious. He admitted to attempting to manufacture meth. He set up a lab in an abandoned shed he found just off the interstate. According to the patient, he added kerosene to his mixture directly before it exploded. In addition to the hand and arm degloving, the patient sustained first, second, and third degree burns to his face, thighs, and abdomen. The flames whooshed through his hair and left a blistered bald patch on the left side of his head. Because the patient screamed instead of gasping, he forced a breath out and saved his lungs from burns.

Soon after the cops left, the patient was heavily sedated and transferred to a hospital with a burn unit.

Uh...Mommy *Meanest*?

I didn't notice when the ambulance entered the bay. Unless I'm bored, looking for a reason, or just happen to catch something out of the corner of my eye, I rarely look at the cameras.

But then a family flooded through the front door and approached the desk and said something that made me look.

"We're here for the ambulance that just came in," gruffly stated a teenage boy.

I looked to two female adults for any indication either would speak on the patient's behalf. Neither of the women seemed too upset. In fact, none of the family members did.

"And what's the name of the patient?" I asked.

The boy answered my question and I informed him the patient was not officially registered with the hospital. Although the patient in the ambulance was likely this family member he sought, I could not allow the family in the back until the patient's identity was confirmed. And, depending on the circumstances and the patient's condition, it was also likely only one family member would be allowed in the back right away: mom.

Nobody in the family took this explanation

very well. They all began berating me but finally walked away from the desk and sat on a wooden bench located by the entrance.

Soon after the family sat down, the patient popped up on the tracking board. The patient was a middle-schooler with a diagnosis of: suicide attempt. It was difficult for me to comprehend the reasons a pre-teen would attempt something so permanent, but it was not my business to theorize.

I looked to the lobby. At two in the morning, the only people there were the patient's family. Each one of the members pecked away on their phones. The teenager mumbled something about not getting decent service and his mother agreed.

As soon as I could access the patient's chart, I called the mother to the desk so I could gather information. She seemed generally disinterested in the process and never asked about the condition of her son. Just as we were wrapping up registration, a nurse emerged from the triage room and asked the patient's mother to come back to her son's room. For the moment, only the mother would be allowed to visit. Because of the circumstances regarding the patient's diagnosis, a police officer and child welfare agent were on the way.

When the nurse explained all of this, the teenage son and the other adult female became irate.

"So he's not even dead? What good is it to try to kill yourself if you fail at that, too?" shouted the teenager.

The nurse and I exchanged worried looks with each other and I think we both fully expected one of the adult women to come unglued and whack the boy upside his head. Instead, they seemed to *agree* with him.

When the nurse disappeared to the back with the patient's mother, the other female and the teenager went to the waiting room. I never really saw them talk to one another.

I finished my work in the patient's chart and walked my paperwork back to the unit clerk.

"You wouldn't believe what that patient's visitor said out there," I whispered.

"Oh," he said in an equal hush, "the nurse told us."

"Yeah, it's crazy."

The unit clerk nodded.

"Did the kid cut himself or what? How'd he try to do it?"

"No," replied the clerk. "I guess he took a bunch of pills he found in the medicine cabinet. Took some heart medication, blood pressure stuff, laxatives. Then, I guess, he washed them all down with a few beers."

"Is it serious right now?"

The clerk shrugged. "They gave him charcoal and an IV in the ambulance. Mom's in there now,

I guess, trying to remember how many pills were in each bottle."

"Wow."

"Yeah."

I returned to the front and was confirmed that the members in the waiting room were the patient's family. The other female was his aunt; the teenager was the patient's brother. I watched the two talk. Occasionally, mom would pop out of the back to go to the parking lot for a smoke. The aunt and teen would join her and light up. I noticed they still did not exhibit worrisome behavior. None of the three were pacing or crying or frequently visiting the restroom. In fact, I would watch them stand in the parking lot and laugh. They'd come through the front doors, still laughing, before retreating to the waiting room and pecking at their phones again.

A police officer and child welfare agent arrived. The patient's mother accompanied the two. Within minutes, I could hear shouting.

"I hate you," echoed throughout the back portion of the ER and through the lobby. A security guard passing through lifted his head toward the commotion before deciding it was time to head back.

I was shocked at the exchange of words. The patient didn't scream them; the mother did as she yelled at her son. She was escorted to the lobby by the police officer and was still grunting and shouting as she was guided to the front door.

"He did this on purpose," she shrieked. "And he wants to say he did it because of how we treat him?"

Upon noticing the scene, the patient's brother jumped up and hurried to the mother's side.

Before I knew it, both family members were yelling at the police officer. I glanced over to the waiting room. Apparently, a rerun of SVU was more important to the aunt than the current events just on the other side of the waiting room glass.

The officer walked the mother and son outside.

While they were in the parking lot, the child welfare agent emerged from the back. She was shaking her head and let out a long sigh.

"That bad, huh?"

"It's something else," she said.

"Talk about dysfunctional," I replied, motioning outside.

"Talk about an understatement," she agreed.

"So now what?"

She shrugged. "I have to go out and make a few calls. There should be a nurse coming out here shortly. You may want to call security and ask them to come out here, just in case."

I nodded and followed her advice. Security suggested it would be a better idea to monitor the situation through the double-sided mirrored wall located just across from the registration desk and perpendicular to the front entrance. They feared the family would become intimidated and further belligerent if they felt we called more officers to the scene.

Our charge nurse walked through the triage room and stood in front of the registration desk.

"They *are* coming back in, right?"

I must have appeared just as puzzled as the thoughts I kept inside my head.

She explained, "They said something about leaving, that they didn't want to be here all night."

"But that's their family," I whispered in surprise.

The nurse shrugged. "Sometimes you just can't reason with people."

The charge nurse waited patiently for the mother and son to come back inside. While they did, the police officer left.

"We're going to go ahead and get him moved upstairs," the nurse explained to the patient's mother.

"But he's fine," protested the brother. "He couldn't go through with it."

"He's stable *now*," the charge nurse replied, "but he ingested several medications that don't normally...*kick in* until many hours later."

"So he could still die?" asked the patient's brother with a hint of excitement in his tone.

"The medication could cause his blood pressure to drop. The pills could interact with one another. There are just so many events that could occur that we feel it's best to move him to our ICU floor for the night."

Mom didn't respond. Instead, she walked over to the waiting room and said to the patient's aunt, "Hey, let me use your phone. Mine's about to die."

The aunt readily handed over her cell phone and the patient's mother began dialing as soon as the device landed in her palm.

She paced the hall in front of the waiting room.

"Hey," I heard her say. "You need to get everyone to the hospital. It's [insert generic name]. They said they're moving him to a different floor because he's dying."

"Hmm," I hummed aloud, without even realizing it.

Our charge nurse waited for the patient's mother to get off the phone, but after several minutes, I think she understood it wasn't really going to happen soon and she needed to get the patient ready to transfer upstairs.

All three family members rode up in the elevator to ICU. I couldn't say I was surprised to see them all walking down the hall and toward the door only a few minutes later.

"Hey," called a nurse. She was nearly out of breath from chasing the family.

The patient's mom stopped, but the teenager and the aunt went outside.

"We've talked and are going home," the mother told the nurse.

I silently watched the blonde-haired nurse. "You're going home?" she exclaimed. She quickly caught herself and said more evenly and calmly, "I thought you might want to stay while he's here. It's possible something could go wrong."

"Can you just call me if he starts to die?" the mother asked, as if the nurse was keeping her from an important meeting.

My mouth fell open.

To my knowledge, the patient was eventually discharged. I couldn't even begin to guess what happened after that.

Early Morning Wood

There's something about the middle of the night that draws people to the hospital. I mean, I know normal people don't wake up from a deep sleep and think, "I know I've had this toe pain for six years now, but *tonight* is when I need to go to the hospital." Sometimes, though, I wonder. And on the night in question, that exact scenario repeated itself in spurts, so much so that the nurses and I could hardly keep up.

But then, without warning, it all stopped. We were grateful for a break from patients and began focusing on the paperwork aspect of the job.

It had been quiet for about an hour and the clock just struck three. I was in the middle of filing away scanned insurance cards when a woman dressed in pink flannel pajama bottoms and a yellow sweatshirt came running inside.

"You have to help him," she shrieked wildly. "You have to help him."

A man walked through the front door. He was shirtless; his tee shirt was wrapped tightly around his right hand.

This happens quite often. A patient will come to the hospital in sheer panic or bring someone along who is panicking, and that 'really bad' injury turns out to be a sliver in the skin from a tin can lid. Because of this gentleman's calm demeanor, I just nodded and pointed to the consent form.

"Let's just calm down," I said to the woman. "I need you to sign for him and—Oh!"

As the man was halfway to the registration desk, I glanced up at him just at the right time to see a thin stream of blood squirt into the air. As I examined him more closely, I noticed he was dripping a trail of blood.

"Let's try to get you back there right now," I said to him.

"My cup holders are full of blood. It just won't stop. I can't get it to stop," he told me without emotion.

I called to the back and quickly told the unit clerk we had someone bleeding profusely.

The man approached the counter.

"Don't touch anything," I hurriedly ordered.

He nodded and stood patiently while I entered his name in the system. As I was doing so, his girlfriend turned to him.

"You have to put more pressure on it," she told him.

The woman reached for his hand with both of hers and clamped down on his palm. If this is done correctly, bleeding should slow.

It wasn't done correctly.

Blood shot out from under every loose crevice

of the tee shirt bandage and spurted in the air like Old Faithful erupting.

"Stop doing that," the man screamed.

A nurse walked through the triage room and stood at the front desk, ready to take the patient. By the look on her face, I believe she was also expecting to be met with a patient presenting a superficial wound, but as soon as he walked around the counter and she saw the blood-soaked shirt and the puddles following him, her lips tightened. She guided the man and woman to the back.

It would only make sense that just after this patient several more would walk in.

"Sit on the bench," I directed hastily. "We can't do anything until this blood is cleaned up. Are you experiencing chest pain or bleeding?"

All three new patients shook their heads and looked at the bloodied lobby with widened eyes.

"There's blood all over your parking lot," one mentioned to me.

A cleaning crew arrived to the lobby within a minute of the operator stat-paging their department. They first cleaned the registration counter and followed that up with a quick mopping so the other patients could register. Nurses, instead of guiding patients through the triage room and to the back, used the double doors and took patients directly to rooms, due to the amount of blood on the triage floor and splattered on the walls. Overall, the cleaning crew spent more than an hour in the lobby and foyer. They had to come back three times because patients arriving, nurses, or I would come across more blood in hard-to-spot places, like smeared on the door, but only visible if it was opened just right; or on the ceilings.

After giving doctors and nurses time to treat the bleeding patient, I traveled to the back to gather more information. I noticed right away that the patient's nurse had changed out of her scrub top and jacket.

"Was it that bad?" I asked her.

She laughed. "When we unwrapped his hand, blood went *everywhere*."

"Did he say what he did?"

The nurse smiled slyly which left me rather excited to enter the patient's room and hear it from his lips.

"Registration," I announced as I knocked and opened the door.

The patient was sitting on the edge of his bed, while his girlfriend was sitting in a burgundy-upholstered chair that was against the far wall.

"You can come in," the man said. He held up his bandaged hand. "They fixed me up."

I could barely fit my cart in the small room because the suture cart was still next to the patient's bed. There was a red plastic bowl atop the cart and it was overflowing with bloody gauze and wrappers.

"How many stitches did you have to get?" I asked.

"Eighteen," he answered proudly.

I nodded.

"So," questioned, "what'd you do?"

"He's an idiot," his girlfriend chimed in with a hard roll of her eyes.

"Well," he replied, "she had gone to bed and she can't sleep with the TV on, so I figured I'd just whittle a little."

"In the dark," the girlfriend added.

"You were whittling in the dark?" I asked with raised brows.

"I've been doing it all my life. Whittling, I mean," the patient told me. "And I just thought I could do it, but..."

"Obviously not, huh?" I asked.

The man laughed. "Yeah, guess not. As soon as I felt the knife go in my skin, I knew it was bad. But I was trying not to wake her up, so I just tried to grab the blanket to stop the bleeding, and I tried to get to the bathroom."

"But he stole all the blankets from me, and then, when he was trying to get to the bathroom, he tripped and fell," said the girlfriend. She didn't seem as amused at the situation as her boyfriend did.

She continued, "He ruined the new comforter I *just* bought. There's blood all over the floor and walls. When I woke up he told me, 'don't turn on the light, babe' but I did, anyway."

The patient nodded. "And she screamed."

"Well," the woman said in annoyance, "there was blood everywhere. It looked like someone got murdered in our bed."

Before the patient left, he promised his girlfriend he would no longer whittle in the dark, perhaps one of the strangest declarations I have ever heard.

When it Rains...

It sometimes seems that for every good thing that happens in the hospital, eight bad things happen to make up for it, almost as if the universe wants to remind us where we are. When working at a hospital, especially in the Emergency Room, a good day can take a bad turn in four seconds. And, usually, when one traumatizing scene is presented, it rarely comes in alone.

I was already having a long day, and I had only been awake for 10 minutes. During my time away from work, I was trying to take care of a stressful situation with a nearby physician's office. Although I presented my insurance card upon registration, the clerk apparently never added it to my file, which meant a bill unexpectedly arrived at my house and the office was demanding $400. In order to remedy the situation, I only had to fax a copy of my insurance card to the office's patient accounts department. So, after throwing on a pair of tattered jeans and a tee shirt, I headed to work.

Boy, was that a mistake.

As I was walking in, I counted five police cars parked in front of the Emergency Room walkway. I instinctively took a deep breath, afraid of what I was about to see.

The lobby was clear when I arrived inside,

which was surprising. It was noon and I didn't see staff members leaving for lunch. The only person at the registration desk was my coworker. I took a quick look to the waiting room. It was packed.

"Are most of those people waiting to be seen?" I asked my coworker.

She groaned and rubbed her eyes.

"No," she replied. "They're all here for someone."

"What's going on?" I motioned to the squad cars outside. "Are they all here for the same room?"

My coworker shook her head. "There's a lot going on right now."

I neared her so I could check out the tracking board.

My brain didn't know where to start, but my mouth blurted out, "A toddler with burns?"

She nodded. "This poor little baby..."

Her eyes teared up and her lips quivered as she choked out the story.

"Her mom was making spaghetti for lunch and went to take the pot off the stove so she could drain it."

"Oh no," I said, anticipating the horror to come.

"Yeah. I guess the little girl was standing behind her, so when the mom turned to walk across the kitchen, she ran into the baby, and—."

The woman sniffled.

"And," she cried, "she dropped a pot of boiling water and hot spaghetti all over the girl. The baby was screaming when they brought her in. Someone said they could hear her down by switchboard. And the mom...The mom is so upset."

"I bet," I replied. "So they're transferring her out?"

"Uh-huh," said my coworker. "They have her sedated right now. The girl's grandparents came in and were yelling at the mom, telling her not to touch the kid until the doctors could take a look. I felt horrible, but I'm glad they told her because all she wanted to do was hold her and touch her."

"Yeah. What did the cops end up saying, do you know?"

A flash of hatred skipped through my coworker's eyes. "The parents said it was an accident, but the cops came in with welfare services because I guess this isn't the first time the baby's been injured like this."

"Really?"

She nodded and motioned to the computer. "When we looked her up, we saw she was just in here last month for a head injury."

"That could've been an accident, too," I said more to myself than to the woman. "But I'm glad they're checking it out."

"They kind of don't know if it's an accident. I'm praying to God it is. The mom was pretty upset about it, so I hope it was an accident."

"Right."

She cleared her throat. "Anyway, they're going to fly her out soon. We're just waiting on the helicopter."

I nodded and walked over to the fax machine.

"And what about those other little girls?"

She gave a hard swallow.

"How can someone even put a child in that situation?" I growled.

See, in addition to the child admitted to the ER for severe burns, three girls, all under the age of nine, were admitted for a diagnosis of: STD check. An adult female and an adult male were also on the board for the same diagnosis.

"And is that guy the dad? Step-dad?" I demanded.

My coworker shook her head and said dryly, "Nope. Brother-in-law to the woman."

"Really?" I exclaimed. "Wow. I don't understand how this stuff happens."

"I guess it wasn't his choice to come in," my coworker explained.

I shook my head. "Disgusting."

She remained calm and tried her best to

display a high level of optimism. "But we're thinking it could be something that wasn't introduced the way we're thinking it was. Like, maybe there wasn't abuse. The uncle said something about having a rash, and the girls all had the same rash."

She rubbed her temples.

"I just don't know what's going on today, and I can't wait for you to come in and relieve me."

I faxed my insurance card and left. With knowledge of how the day had gone for my coworker, the last thing I wanted to do was go back to work that evening.

The painful truth is healthcare workers do witness horrific accidents on a daily basis. For some, it is difficult to think beyond the sadness and anger that accompany these events. It takes a strong person to see pure pain in a patient's eyes, to see a patient's family experiencing fear, and then to go on about our day as if it's all okay. But we have to do that to bring comfort to the next family. Nobody in this industry can escape the eventual viewing of utter devastation and loss. We often fall asleep at night, praying our actions and words positively impacted a patient's experience, and we often catch ourselves thinking about a patient we encountered years ago. Caring, praying, hoping, crying...That is healthcare. Despite all the bad things we see, we still wake up and hope for the best for the new day.

Friendly Reminder:

Cost of a pregnancy test at a nearby Dollar Tree: $1 + tax.

Cost of a pregnancy test in the Emergency Room: more than you'll ever want to know.

Just the Tip

On a slow evening shift, a woman calmly walked to the desk.

"Can we help you?" my coworker asked.

The woman nodded and gave her name and date of birth.

"And what seems to be the problem tonight?"

"A cat bit my finger off," the patient replied without blinking.

"*A cat bit your finger off?*" repeated my coworker in surprise. Even I raised my head. The patient was calmer than the waters of a stagnant pond. There was absolutely no expression of pain in her actions, words, or exuding from her eyes.

The patient lifted her left hand to the counter to display her towel-wrapped ring finger.

"Yep," she answered. "It just took my finger right off."

"Was it your cat?" my coworker questioned.

"It sounds more like a leopard," I joked to another coworker under my breath.

"No," said the woman, shaking her head. "I was taking trash to the can in the alley and there was this pretty yellow cat on top of the can. So I started petting it and it let me. Then, all the sudden—you know, like cats do—I guess it decided that was enough. It just bit my finger off and ran away. My neighbor saw the whole thing. She's parking her car and will bring the rest of my finger with her in a minute or so."

My coworker gasped. "You brought your finger with you?"

"Well...*yeah,*" the patient laughed. "It'd be nice if they could sew it back on. They do it in the movies, right? I mean, do you think they'll be able to do it here?"

"I-I don't know," my coworker stammered.

An elderly woman came running in a waddle through the front door. She was waving an ice-filled Tupperware container high above her head and shouted, "I have the finger. Here it is, so you can save her finger."

I couldn't help but to laugh.

The triage nurse was called and when she called the patient, she looked strangely to the diagnosis and then back to the woman.

"A cat bit your finger?"

"Off," the patient corrected. "It bit my finger off."

"Your cat?"

The patient told her story all over again before going to the back, where I'm sure she told it several more times to other doctors and nurses. From what I understand, she remained collected during her entire stay, despite the fact that a cat, indeed, bit her finger down to the bone. Luckily for her, doctors were able to reattach the chomped digit. Nurses remarked how she never exhibited even an ounce of pain.

Now, after dealing with this patient, I couldn't help but to think back to a group of macho men in the ER a few months before the cat incident. That incident went a completely different direction.

I was working part of a day shift and seven men rushed through the front door, huddled around an eighth man—who was sobbing loudly—in the center. Most of the men were six feet tall, at least, and all but one were beefy men with big bellies and long beards. Three of the men were wearing camouflage jumpsuits.

"He needs a doctor," several of the men were shouting.

"Okay," I cooed, "let's just calm down. I need one person to tell me what's happened."

The men looked to one another before visually cuing one of the camo-clad men to answer my question.

"He, uh...Okay, so we were hunting and messing around and I don't know how it happened, but he somehow shot the tip of his finger off."

"And they couldn't find it," the patient screamed through his cries. "Please help me. I don't want to bleed to death."

When I asked for the patient's name and date

of birth, another one of the men from the group stepped forward and demanded, "We need to skip this part for now. This is the ER and this man can't wait."

"Sir," I asked the patient, "do you have your hand wrapped right now?"

He nodded and lifted his hand to the counter. Around the tip of his index finger were three paper towels. The outer paper towel was spotless. The wound obviously wasn't bleeding enough to soak through the wrapping.

"Now," I explained, "there's nobody in front of you after the nurse finishes triaging the patient she has back there right now. I need to ask you and your friends to take a seat in the waiting room for a few minutes. It's possible that another nurse from the back will come out here for you. It shouldn't take too long either way. Two friends can go to the room with you."

"I can't sit down," the patient argued. "You need to tell them this is an emergency."

"I'll call and let them know you're here," I said.

Before I could pick up the phone, a nurse walked through triage and asked, "Is there a problem here?"

All eight of the men started to speak at once.

"One at a time," the nurse said. "Which of you is the patient?"

The man in the center of the group raised his non-injured hand and was taken to the back with two of his friends, while the other five men stood at the desk and explained they had meant to spend the day hunting and hiding from their wives.

In the middle of our talk, I heard the patient shriek shrilly.

According to the nurse, the bullet from the patient's gun grazed his fingertip and took a shallow chunk from the end of his finger, but it was nothing that wouldn't heal. A doctor from the back stated the man would probably have a slight permanent indention on his fingertip, but the bullet didn't even come close to the man's fingernail. While I thought the man was receiving a shot to numb the area, perhaps to saw down bone, what actually caused him to scream was the burning sensation of an IV of saline flowing through his veins.

These two incidents are proof that severity of wounds cannot be measured by how much pain the patient seems to be in (or doesn't seem to be in). I'm not sure what happened to either patient, but I can bet the woman won't be petting stray cats for a while, and the hunter will probably be a bit more careful with firearms in the future.

What Hospital Workers Want to Tell You

　　* Waiting can sometimes be a good sign. If you are sitting in the waiting room with a knife sticking out of your heart, are rolling around on the floor in a pool of your own vomit, or you pass out from the pain you've experienced from that throbbing in your right side, eh, it's probably *not* really a good sign for you. However, we wish we could tell you to calm down. We understand your ailment must be 'really bad' to make you decide to visit the Emergency Room, but if you are waiting, that usually means someone in worse shape than you is seeing a doctor or nurse right now. Events like shootings, motor vehicle accidents, and chest pains have power to impact the waiting period. If you are waiting to be seen, it usually means we don't think you're going to code or die while you're doing it. If you feel angry that you have been waiting for ten minutes, think about how long those ten minutes must be for the eight-year-old daughter of a man who's been brought in because someone shot him in the heart and doctors are doing everything they can to save that man's life. Waiting isn't always a bad thing.

　　* You mean to tell me you've had a rock

lodged under your skin for four years, but, even though you're not suffering or feeling the slightest bit of discomfort, you've decided to come to the ER *now* and then complain that there are 12 patients in front of you?

* Find a primary doctor. And when you do, visit *that* office. We understand some situations call for immediate attention, but coming to the ER for a runny nose at six in the morning when you know the doctor's office opens in two hours is going a bit overboard.

* Answering single to marital status doesn't mean your boyfriend is hitting on the nurse or the registration person. It just means you're not married. Oh, wait. That causes problems, too. I can't tell you how many fights the marital status question has caused.

* On that note, we know it's stressful and you're comfortable around us, but family drama is awwwwwwkwaaaaard.

* Nope, this isn't *House*. We probably don't have a doctor here capable of diagnosing your mystery illness. Furthermore, the odds are slim to none that you have (or will *ever* have) a mystery illness.

* Thanks for telling me that WebMD diagnosed you with CHF and a ruptured spleen, but your EKG concluded your heart is fine and it's probably indigestion from the eight chili dogs with extra jalapenos you admitted to chowing down two hours ago.

* Learn your spouse's social security number. Learn your child's social security number. Learn your *own* social security number. It can save your loved one's or your life, especially in cases where you've visited the hospital before but your previous chart can't be found by name. If you don't know your child's birthday, learn it. Know which medicines you're taking. The suggestions here may appear to be common sense, but we see more clueless people walk through the front doors than anyone could imagine. It can mean the difference between receiving a medicine that interacts poorly with one you're taking. It can mean your insurance claim won't be handled properly. Learn your information. Learn your family's information.

* We're not being mean when we won't let you back to see your friend or family member. Visitors are often restricted from rooms if the patient is undergoing certain tests or exams. Some Emergency Rooms have limitations on the number of visitors that may enter the patient's room. There

are a number of reasons why someone may not be able to visit a patient. Some of these may directly pertain to your friend or family member. Other reasons, however, may have nothing to do with you or the person you wish to visit. There are times when a patient codes or all hell breaks loose in the back, and during these times, some charge nurses lock down the ER to keep hall traffic to a minimum. It's usually not personal.

* I once went nine hours without peeing and a woman five-months-pregnant had to go 10 hours without eating because we were so busy none of us could find time to take a break. We're all tired, overworked, and underpaid. Face it, you probably often feel the same way, right? There is a difference between being snappy because you're in pain versus being flat-out rude because you think the doctors, nurses, and other hospital members should be at your every beck and call. This isn't a restaurant. This isn't a fun house. We're all here to make sure you're healthy and to hopefully make sure you don't die.

* It takes time for emergency vehicles to reach the hospital. Then, after the ambulance arrives, it takes time to wheel the patient inside. After EMTs help nurses situate the new patient on a hospital bed, the patient's name and date of birth is most likely given to a unit clerk or registration clerk. The patient then has to be registered and certain documents have to be given to nursing staff. Doctors and nurses will enter the patient's room and attempt to prioritize the situation. This all takes time. It may not be possible for you to enter the patient's room right away. Under certain circumstances, a staff member may invite you straight back. If you know pertinent medical information that may have not been relayed to EMTs, notify someone immediately. If you know the patient cannot communicate, indicate this. It will help us take care of the patient and it could get you to the room faster.

* If you're able to tell me your entire life story, you're obviously not *that* short of breath. I also saw you in the waiting room, eating a bag of Doritos and laughing with your friend, before the nurse walked by and you suddenly became the sickest, loudest person waiting to be seen.

* "I tried [random pain medicine], but it didn't work. The only thing that works for me is a double dose of Dilaudid." You don't have to be a nurse to hear this several times per night. It's one thing to say this *after* a nurse or doctor offers a first choice of medicine, but please keep in mind that when you say this before you're offered medication, it makes you sound like a drug seeker.

****I would like to add an after-publication

note to clarify this. Chronic pain sufferers, this doesn't apply to you. Doctors are here to HELP you. Unfortunately, we see a lot of people with non-chronic injuries or hospital-hoppers who come in and ask for medication by name before even telling us where the pain is.

* Prioritize and keep it in a nutshell until you're with a nurse or doctor. Registration clerks don't need to hear every last detail about your illness or your day. Tell us the major problems first if you want to get in faster.

* Ambulances aren't taxis. It's not cool to call an ambulance because you have a headache, suddenly 'feel better,' and ask EMS or the ambulance driver to drop you off at your friend's house located in the next town. (In this town, a private ambulance service hires drivers— paramedics handle patients with this service. There's no offense meant, just the way that agency runs things. We simply have a company with only drivers and then another service where the drivers are also EMTs/medics.)

* 'I'm really sick' doesn't tell me a whole lot. Neither does 'It's really bad.' Yeah, you should keep to the point, but give us a little more to go on so we know where to start.

* Arriving on an ambulance doesn't necessarily mean you'll be taken straight to the back. On a crazy shift when we were so backed up that the shortest waiting time was three hours, a frequent flyer (a patient who visits the ER so often staff members know this person by name and can often guess the patient's diagnosis) called an ambulance because her toe hurt. EMTs were instructed to place the patient in a wheelchair, where she was to wait to be seen. The patient was irate and spent her entire waiting period attempting to get taken straight back. Some of her complaints during the waiting time included her claiming she had chest pain, her faking passing out and dramatically falling to the floor (she miraculously recovered when she realized it wasn't helping her), and forcing herself to cough until she vomited.

* Get off the phone when we need to talk to you. Your conversation about football can wait if you're really claiming you're feeling a 10 on the pain scale.

* If you're being difficult and threaten to leave because you're not getting your way by throwing your hissy fit, BYE. We are here to help you feel your best, not to kiss your butt and serve you dinner.

* Nice try on noticing we're super busy and telling me you suddenly have chest pain. Bet you didn't think they'd do an EKG in triage and send you back to the waiting room when it came back normal, did you?

* Don't tell the registration person you have chest pain, but then tell the nurse you don't.

Having a Bad Day

An intoxicated man visited the ER with dried blood spread over his lips and chin. He held a yellow dish towel in his hand and occasionally to his sideways nose.

"I think I broke my nose," he told the registration clerk.

Yes, the man's doctor confirmed, he did break his nose.

The patient wasn't in the ER too terribly long.

When it came time for him to leave, he thanked the registration clerks and went on about his way. As he approached the front door, it was easy to tell he was going to the wrong side. Although there are three plates of glass across the opening and one would *think* the door opens from both ends, it only opens from one, and it wasn't the end the man was nearing.

Now, this man was staggering about and walking briskly, determined to get back home. He was in such a hurry and had such faith that the door would open that he didn't bother slowing down.

The man's face bounced off the glass and he dropped his discharge papers on the floor. When he turned to the registration desk, his hands were already over his nose and blood was pouring through his loose fingertips.

"I think I broke my nose again," he said in a muffled voice.

Yes, he did.

Hunting Accident

On a long overnight shift, a man walked through the front door and approached the registration desk.

"I'm gonna need some help getting my brother out of the truck," he said to me.

I nodded. "I'll call for help. Can you tell me what brings him here tonight?"

The man seemed confused. "Uh...A truck."

I smiled. "I mean, is he sick? Is he having chest pain?"

That's when I smelled the beer seeping from the man's pores.

"Oh, no. The dumbass fell out of a tree."

"Uh, okay."

I called the back and notified them that help was needed. One male tech and a female nurse went outside and wheeled in another man. This man's face was covered in scratches and he was breathing loudly and rhythmically, like a woman in labor. The tightly-laced black boot on his right foot was turned completely to the right, with the toe of the boot facing security's office.

"I thought about taking his shoe off," the patient's brother told the nurses, "but I thought the pressure might be the only thing keeping his whole foot from swelling up."

"How did he do this?" the nurse asked.

The brother replied, "He fell."

I stayed up front and registered a few patients presenting cold symptoms. Then, after about an hour, enough time had passed that x-ray and other departments were able to get in and out of the patient's room to perform tests and exams.

I headed to the back and rolled my cart to the patient's room.

"Good luck," whispered a passing nurse as she emerged from his room.

Those aren't words you ever want to hear from your coworker when you work in a hospital.

"Oh God," I mumbled.

The patient's room did not have a door, so instead I knocked on the door frame and pulled the teal curtain open.

"Go away," said the patient. "I'm not guilty of anything."

I raised my brows.

The patient's brother was standing on the other side of the room with his back up against a counter.

"Shut up," he said to the patient. "Answer her questions so we can get out of here."

As I started asking the patient initial demographic questions, such as his marital status and ethnicity, he gruffed and grumbled. But he answered them, and he didn't hesitate answering me when I asked for his address.

When I reached the accident screen, however, the patient decided he didn't want to talk to me anymore. To express this, he called me every name in the book in a strand of two seconds, I do believe.

"If you don't stop I'm going to come over there and break the other ankle," his brother warned. "Look, I'll answer for him. He's just afraid he's going to get in trouble and lose his job."

"So what happened?" I asked the brother.

The man shook his head and rubbed his eyes. "We were out late, deer hunting and drinking. This genius decides to drink so much he can't stand on his own, so he used his shotgun as a crutch and tried to take a leak from twenty feet up in an oak tree."

"Hmmm," I replied.

"Yeah," said the brother. "And everything was fine. Oh, you know, till the gun gave way and he fell out of the tree stand. And see, the gun landed upright on the ground, so the barrel caught him in the back like those skateboarding idiots you see in those videos when they hit railings."

"Ouch," I added.

"See, that's not even the bad part," the brother continued. "His pants are down. His junk is all hanging out. He hits the gun. And then, he landed on his ankle. For a split second, I heard the crack. But then I heard the shotgun go off."

"Well," I said, "I'm glad nobody was hurt by the gun."

"Didn't get shot," the patient said, "but I sure did piss myself."

The patient's break wasn't as bad as he thought. The injury was set and the man was fitted with a cast and given a pair of crutches—the kind that wouldn't shoot if the patient dropped them as he was falling out of a tree.

The patient's last words to me were: "I hope I can still hunt while taking hydrocodone."

Curl Up and Watch a Movie

A family member worked in the registration desk when I was younger, and I will never forget the story he had to tell one night.

According to the family member, a patient arrived at the ER registration desk with a rather odd complaint: his hand was stuck in a VCR.

In addition to the patient's complaint, he asked if he could get a blanket. He was cold, and that made sense, since he was also buck naked.

According to the patient, he disrobed and planned to watch a few adult flicks and...ahem...enjoy himself while watching. When the VCR started eating the tape, the man pressed stop and then attempted to eject the tape from the device. When this wouldn't work, the man stuck his hand inside the VCR and tried to pull out the tape. This is when his hand became stuck.

Nobody really knows why the man decided to come in naked, but at the time my family member told the story, he thought the man's confession of doing drugs had a lot to do with it.

An Eye for an Eye

A frantic mother scurried to the registration desk one evening. She was crying and holding her small son at a strange angle, careful not to apply pressure to the child's diapered bottom or the back of his upper thighs.

She told me her son's information through tears.

"What's going on right now?" I asked. "Does he have a diaper rash?"

"I wish," she sniffled.

The patient's grandmother was standing next to mom.

"You need to tell them what really happened," grandma urged her daughter.

"I let my fiancé babysit and when I came home, he had beaten my son so hard that both of his butt cheeks are purple."

"And there are these thin, red and purple welts down his back, too. After flipping out on the guy, he finally told us he whipped the baby with electrical wire."

The child wasn't even two years old. I felt sick to my stomach.

"Have you notified the authorities?" I asked.

Grandma and mom both nodded.

"But he ran," mom said. "The cops went over to his apartment but said they can't do anything until they find him."

Grandma said, "They told us to come here. An officer is on the way and someone from CPS has to come so they can take pictures."

I notified triage and the patient was taken to the triage room. That didn't last long. The baby screamed as soon as he was touched by the stranger and the nurse concluded the injuries were so severe that the child needed to be moved to the back immediately.

According to nurses in the back, the child was beaten so hard and for so long that his back had swollen in spots to the size of a grapefruit, and he was missing skin on his back, buttocks, and thighs. An officer and child welfare agent did visit the patient's room to document the abuse and spoke to the patient's mother about what actions to take next.

When I entered the patient's room to gather more information, the mother was screaming into her cell phone. Judging by the harsh words and threats, there was no doubt in my mind she was speaking to her fiancé.

"I'm never marrying that man," she shouted to her mother as the call ended.

"Good," grandma replied. "Because if he can do this to a child, just think of what he'll try to do to you. He's a coward."

The patient was eventually released and a few shifts had passed.

On a busy evening shift, two men approached the counter. One of the men had a bath towel wrapped around his arm and his face was bloody. Both of his eyes were swollen and ringed in purple and black bruises, and his bottom lip was busted open. As he breathed through his mouth, I noticed one of his front canine teeth was missing and the rest of his teeth were stained in red.

"What happened here?" I asked.

"I, uh, got my arm stuck in a barbed wire fence and am cut up pretty bad."

"That's all?" I questioned skeptically.

His friend nodded. "He said that's what happened, so that's what happened. He needs to be seen by a doctor now, before he bleeds to death."

We had at least nine patients waiting to be seen, and the back was filled up to the point that there were no empty beds. I explained the situation to the patient but assured him I would notify the charge nurse.

I sent the patient to the waiting room. During the wait time, his friend approached the counter several times, demanding to know what was taking so long and why the two weren't being treated accordingly. I explained the bed situation again, but neither of the men were satisfied. Fifteen minutes passed before the two men were walked to the back.

Shortly after the patient's arrival, a female approached the desk. I knew I recognized her from someplace, but I couldn't put my finger on it.

"My fiance's back there," she motioned behind me. "And I need to go see him."

I called to the back to make sure the patient could have another visitor, to which his nurse allowed. I unlocked the double doors for the woman and she disappeared to the back.

When I went back to gather information from the patient, the female was gripping his hand and kissing his forehead. Doctors had already visited the room and the patient's bloody towel was on the floor. On his arm, from his wrist to his elbow, doctors had placed nine staples to close a long, shallow gash.

The patient's fiancée answered most of the questions, but when it came to the accident screen, the patient's male friend answered.

"We were out messing around in the country and he got his arm stuck in a barbed wire fence."

He was firm with his reply and his tone suggested I left well enough alone, so I thanked the three for cooperating and I left the room.

"So," asked the charge nurse as I passed, "what do you think of that situation?"

"I kind of wonder what *really* happened," I answered.

"You don't remember the woman in there, do you?"

I shook my head. "She looks so familiar, but I don't know who she is."

"Remember that abused baby last week?"

And then it hit me.

"Oh my," I exclaimed in a loud whisper. "That's the mom."

The head nurse nodded. "And you weren't here when the rest of her family came last week, were you?"

"No," I answered.

"Well," explained the charge nurse, "that other guy is the woman's brother."

My eyes widened.

It all made sense.

A Hairy Situation

A first-time mom brought her six-day old son to the ER one evening. She was crying and went through eight tissues just as she gave me her child's name and date of birth.

"I just know I messed up his circumcision," she blubbered. "And now he's going to grow up and people are going to make fun of his penis. He's never going to be able to find a girlfriend or get married or get a good job."

I bit my lip and tried to take a second to think. It was hard not to laugh.

"What exactly is going on, mom?" I asked her. "Is the site bleeding?"

She shook her head. "His penis is like this big," she said, as she held up a fist. "And it's purple. I don't know what I did to mess him up so bad already."

"Let's just try to calm down for now. We have a few pretty great doctors and nurses here, and they'll probably have him fixed right up."

I walked around the counter to guide the mother to the waiting room. She picked up her son's car seat from the floor. He wasn't crying. In fact, he seemed content with life as he gazed upward.

When I returned to the desk, the triage nurse was gathering the baby's paperwork.

"Swollen penis?" she asked.

I nodded. "And mom is freaking out, so just a warning."

"Thanks," she replied.

The mother and child were in triage for a little over three minutes. Six minutes after being taken to the back, I noticed the patient had been discharged.

"That was quick," I said to myself.

I looked up to see the new mother leaving. She lugged her baby's car seat in her left hand.

"Is everything okay?" I called to her.

Mom turned and approached the counter. Her face was as red as the skin around her eyes.

"I'm so embarrassed," she laughed nervously.

"Why?"

"His circumcision is fine."

"That's good, then," I smiled. "Was it just normal swelling?"

"No," she said. She leaned in and whispered to me, "They found a strand of my hair wrapped around his wee-wee. It was cutting off his circulation."

"Me and my husband were arguing and I tried to kick him as he was leaving, but I missed and fell off the porch."

– A patient, on how she sustained an ankle and tailbone injury.

Repeat Trip

A male and female entered the ER and both wished to be seen.

The female's diagnosis was: feels like she's going to have a seizure, while her boyfriend's diagnosis was: stomach pains and grumbling.

Doctors and nurses examined the *interesting* couple and concluded the woman, who admitted she never actually had a seizure, was fine, and her boyfriend was simply hungry.

Staff members advised the female to rest for the remainder of the evening and directed her boyfriend to a local grocery store.

Both of the patients were back at my desk within an hour.

"You're back," I chirped to the female. "Did you guys forget something?"

The woman shook her head. "I ate glass."

"You ate glass?" I repeated.

She nodded. "See, we went to get groceries. We bought some mustard, beef jerky..."

I zoned out as the woman used her fingers to count every item she and her boyfriend purchased.

"So we bought twenty things," she told me.

"Okay...So how did you eat the glass?"

"We were walking home and I was carrying the bag with the jar of mustard. And I tripped. The bag fell and the jar broke."

"Okay."

"So we got home and I went to eat beef jerky. And I think the glass cut the beef jerky wrapper open."

"Was the wrapper open when you went to eat the beef jerky?" I asked.

She shook her head. "I think it cut through the side. Now I can feel the glass cutting my throat and I can feel it shredding my stomach. I think I'm going to bleed to death."

I stared at the patient for a brief second.

'Possibly ingested glass,' I typed as her complaint. I didn't know what else to type to give the back ER staff a warning as to what they would be dealing with.

After a few scans and tests, doctors told the patient they believed she was okay. They were almost positive the patient did not ingest glass. The patient and her boyfriend left again and I never saw them again.

"Yeah, I drank a lot last night and this morning I woke up with a headache. I've also been puking, feel dizzy, can't think about food without feeling sick, and I'm tired. I don't know what's happening to me."

– A patient, describing her ailment. She was clinically diagnosed with what modern medicine professionals like to call a 'hangover.'

Read the Instructions

An elderly man approached the registration desk and placed a silver cardboard box on the counter.

"Can I help you?" I asked.

"Yeah," he nodded. "See, I've been throwing up quite a bit lately, so I went over to my doctor this morning and he gave me some of these pills."

"Okay," I replied.

"He told me to use one pill every four hours."

"Okay."

"Well," he said, grabbing at the package and removing one of the white pills, "I don't usually complain—wasn't brought up that way. But, ma'am, these pills get all mushy in my mouth and they taste foul. I think there either must be something wrong with them, or maybe I can just get one of your people see me and write a new prescription, given my doctor is closed this late?"

The man smashed the pill he was holding between his fingers and it hit me at once.

"Sir," I asked, "can I see that box?"

He handed me the carton and as soon as I saw the wording on the label, I laughed.

"Sir," I explained, "these are suppositories."

"Well, I'll be damned," he exclaimed. "That sure explains a lot."

Highly intoxicated man: "Is this where I need to go if I have an emergency and need help?"

Coworker: "Yes."

Highly intoxicated man: "Okay, just checking. I'll come back later if I need help."

Full of Crap

During a shift so busy that nurses were seeing patients in makeshift 'rooms' set up in the ambulance bay, a patient came to the registration desk. I was called in on my day off to help my coworkers keep up with the patients for half a shift, so I had not yet clocked in and had not yet removed my coat. As I was placing my purse on the counter, I listened to one of my coworkers as she registered the patient at the desk. Everything seemed fine, at first. But when it came to directing the patient to the waiting room, the man became irate.

"But I just told you I have a sore throat. You're *really* making me wait for that? There must be at least fifteen people in front of me."

"Sir, I apologize for your wait, but we're busy right now. It is possible several people will be discharged from the back and the line will move a bit faster, but right now we have no choice other than ask patients to wait."

I watched as the man shook his head in irritation. He didn't say another word, though. Instead, he did walk to the waiting room, where he took a seat in the center of the room.

Five minutes after the man sat down, I noticed a few patients had gotten up from their seats and had taken to standing in the hallway. I didn't think too much of it.

Ten minutes later, another patient from the waiting room walked out and approached the desk. I fully expected the patient to ask just how long she had until she was seen by a doctor.

"Can I help you?" I asked the woman.

She leaned in. "I'm sorry to complain, but the man in there, in the middle of the room, keeps opening his colostomy bag. It's really bothering a lot of people."

"Thank you for letting me know," I answered. "I'll let someone know. We'll definitely try to get this handled."

As the woman walked away, I picked up the phone and called security.

"Was there a problem with that woman?" one of the guards asked.

I shook my head at the double-sided mirror. "Did you see that guy we just sent to the waiting room a few minutes ago?"

"Yeah. What's up?"

"Well, that woman said the man we just registered keeps opening his colostomy bag. I don't know if you can maybe say something to him or what, but I'm guessing our wait times are at an hour or more right now."

The guard paused. "I'll try to say something to make him stop."

"Thanks."

One of our security guards emerged from their hidden office and walked to the waiting room. I watched as the guard spoke to the patient.

"And I said it was an accident," I heard the patient scream.

The guard returned to the desk and started to tell me what the patient had said, but I told him I heard everything.

"So," the guard said, "we'll just go from here."

"Yeah."

Another patient was at the desk five minutes later.

"This guy keeps opening his bag," complained another man at the registration desk. "Look, I understand some of us have problems, but he keeps laughing when he does it. My daughter is here to be seen, but I'm going to have to take her somewhere else if you can't make this man stop. My daughter is getting sick to her stomach from the smell."

"Okay," I answered. "I'll go ahead and see if we can get it taken care of."

I made another call to security.

"More problems?" the guard asked.

I nodded. "Same guy, same problem."

This time, both security officers approached the patient. They issued a second warning to the man.

"You can't kick me out of here," he yelled. "You can't make me leave if I need medical attention."

It was clear several other waiting patients wanted to respond, but nobody did.

"And we're not asking you to leave," one of the security guards said. "But if this continues we will have to move you to a different location. We can see you on camera, and we see that you're doing this intentionally."

The patient screamed a few more times. Security warned the gentleman that if he opened his bag one more time, they would take action to move him to a consultation room. There would be no television, no magazines, and he still would not be seen until it was his turn.

Security returned to the registration desk and stood behind my coworkers and me.

Although the patient had been warned, he apparently did not care.

A third patient approached the desk ten minutes later and complained. She then left the hospital in disgust.

"That's it," one of the security guards announced. He motioned for his coworker to follow. "Come on. Let's get him out of the waiting room and to the consultation room."

I watched as security talked to the patient.

The man stood and shouted, "Well I'm leaving, anyway."

A few people applauded. A few people cheered. But nobody tried to stop him.

All in the Name of Vanity

I was working an overnight shift when a young man carried a young woman through the front door. She was wearing teeny-tiny mesh shorts and no shoes. Blood was running down the woman's leg from a shallow gash in her upper thigh.

"What happened?" I asked.

The man laughed and sat the woman in the chair.

"It's not funny," she snapped at him. She then looked to me. "I fell and cut my leg open on the corner of a concrete stair."

The man laughed harder and louder.

"Come on up here and let's get you registered," I directed.

"Why don't you tell her the truth while you're at it?" the man asked the woman.

"That *was* the truth," she growled.

"Yeah, for why you were in the hospital last week."

"I'm confused," I declared. "What's going on right now?"

The man looked to me and said, "She *did* fall last week. We took her to another hospital and the doctor there gave her stitches."

"Okay," I answered.

"Don't do this," the woman begged.

"But my genius girlfriend here decided she was going to tear her stitches out tonight."

I glanced to the woman as if to ask her if there was any truth to the story.

She sighed. "I was invited to a pool party happening Saturday."

It was after midnight.

"Saturday?" I asked. "Like, tonight?"

She nodded and continued, "Well, I couldn't go with my leg stitched up. I mean, I'd look horrible."

"Uh, okay."

I took the woman's information and registered her.

"So you really tore your stitches out?" I questioned.

"Yes," she replied.

"She used a steak knife to do it," her boyfriend added.

"What was I supposed to do?" the woman shouted at her boyfriend. "You want me to have pictures taken with nasty black stitches on my leg? Do you know how disgusting and stupid that would have looked?"

He shook his head in disbelief. "I'm sure you could've turned sideways like you do in all the rest of your pictures."

"You know I have to turn left. I just don't look as good when I turn right."

The man scoffed. "Well, it was a *really* great idea to tear your stitches out."

I had to agree with the man.

I sent the patient to the waiting room and went to the back to explain to the triage nurse what the patient had done. A few doctors and nurses overheard me and laughed.

Unfortunately, for the patient's ever-so-important look, she received *more* stitches to close the wound she opened when she cut out her stitches eight days earlier than they were supposed to be removed. As she was leaving the hospital, I heard her tell her boyfriend he ruined her life and now she couldn't go to the party because she would "look like crap."

"A man had come in to complain of rectal pain. It turns out he had a 'D' battery stuck in his butt. They had to take him to surgery to get it out because he actually pushed it up further and further when he tried to get it out."

—My coworker, when I asked if he could remember the first strange thing he heard or saw during his employment.

Blink and It's Gone

A female patient showed up with her husband and tearfully asked to be seen.

"I feel like my bones are on fire," she said.

When triage asked how long the woman had been experiencing the pain, she said she experienced the pain for months, but she finally got a new job with good insurance, so now she could afford to visit a doctor or ER. She said she understood she could have come to the ER when she didn't have insurance, but she and her husband were barely making it as it was, and she couldn't afford another bill. It was a disheartening explanation.

This patient was in the back portion of the ER for more than five hours before she was diagnosed with a rare bone condition. Her illness likely grew in strength as it went on undetected for years, and by the time she started experiencing pain, it had taken control. Doctors recommended that the patient be sent upstairs for observation. The patient declined, citing a long work day the next day. She felt she could not let the company down, and she was fearful of losing her job. This patient signed AMA (against medical advice) release forms and thanked everyone for the kindness and help she received.

A few hours later, the patient was back at the registration desk. This time, her husband had situated her in one of the extra-wide wheelchairs. She curled up sideways in the chair but kept her right leg dangled over the side. She was in excruciating pain and sobbed.

This time around, the patient said she bumped her shin against her coffee table. She said it was something she had done a thousand times before, but this time she felt as if she had been shot with a bazooka.

Doctors examined the patient and concluded she fractured her tibia. They suggested the fracture went hand-in-hand with the patient's disease and again recommended that she be transferred to another floor for observation. This time, the patient did not argue as much. She expressed regret in having to call in to work, but she accepted she needed the rest after everything she'd been through that day.

The next night, the patient's husband passed through the ER to visit his wife's room.

"I hope your wife is doing better," I said to him.

He stopped and shook his head. "They say now that she has some kind of infection caused by the break."

By the next time I saw the husband, which was the next night—two days after the patient was seen in the ER—he told us his wife was being moved to our Hospice floor because the infection had spread to her blood and there was nothing professionals could do to heal her.

It was shocking to hear such news. Several patients come to the ER for ailments that seem insignificant, only to be diagnosed with lung masses or uterine cancer hours later. But to see a seemingly-healthy patient come through the ER and end up in Hospice two days later is a feeling like no other.

There were two adults at the desk as the first round of visitors to the patient's room.

"Expect more," they told me. "We're having a party to celebrate her life."

I nodded and expected a handful of visitors.

As the night progressed, more than 50 visitors arrived to visit with the patient. We directed delivery guys from every restaurant in town to the patient's room, and even most of the visitors brought snacks and soft drinks. Registration called to the floor to check in with the floor nurses. Although it was a sad situation, the patient was appreciative of her friends and family lending emotional support.

The patient expired the next day. Her husband said she held on long enough for her mother to fly in from Orlando and visit.

College Crazies

Because there is a college in this town, we have our fair share of students coming in for treatment. Here are few reasons local college students have visited the ER:

* Five chest pain complaints from young adults ranging from 18 to 22-years-old came in back to back. We finally learned (from another young patient having a panic attack) that finals were the next day.

* "My roommate is black, and with all this stuff about Ebola, I think I need to be checked to make sure she didn't give it to me."

* A young man came in and demanded a test on his new bar of soap. He swore his roommates put drops of poison on the soap because each time he washed with it, he broke out in an itchy rash. What was more surprising is that his *mother* then called us, demanding the same thing.

* A female arrived and asked to be seen. When I asked her what seemed to be the problem, she said there was nothing wrong, but she was

hoping a trip to the ER would get her an extension on her paper that was due in eight hours.

* A teen patient arrived via ambulance for a complaint of: itchy finger. It was a mosquito bite.

* Another teen arrived via ambulance for a suicide attempt called in by her roommate. "I really wasn't going to kill myself," the patient told me. "I just wanted something good to post on Facebook to get this guy's attention." The patient was released after a psychiatric evaluation and the determination that the ten pills she ingested were multivitamins.

* Two young women with tiny baby bumps approached the registration desk with a third flat-bellied friend in tow. The girls claimed they made a pact to get pregnant at the same time, but they 'knew' something was wrong with the third girl's pregnancy when she experienced vaginal bleeding. When the patient was alone in the exam room, with her friends in the waiting room, she confessed that she never actually wanted to get pregnant, but she felt if she didn't lie about it to the other girls, they wouldn't want to be friends with her. She said she was able to hide her period for three months, but this time one of the other girls walked in while the patient was using the restroom. Instead of 'fessing up immediately, the patient lied to the

other girls and said she must be having a miscarriage. I'm not sure what happened when the patient left or if she ever confessed the real reason she now had a bill from the Emergency Room.

Children are the Future

I had just gotten to work and there were several patients in the back, but registration only needed to gather more information from two of those patients to complete their charts. I headed straight back. By the time I could start up the laptop on the registration cart, there was only one patient left to visit.

The patient in question was a 19-year-old female with a complaint of: hand laceration.

I figured the story would be something boring. She was probably trying to cut an apple or something equally lame. Most of the diagnoses across the tracking board were the typical ones: cold symptoms, headache, vomiting. I just couldn't imagine that the patient's injury could possibly add any spice to the evening.

"Registration," I announced.

I entered the room to see the patient in bed. Five other teenagers stood around the room. Only two visitors are usually allowed in a patient's room, but I brushed it off as nobody cared.

I took the young lady's information and couldn't wait to get out of the room.

"Okay," I said. "How did you cut yourself?"

She blushed.

"I've heard it all," I said. "Were you cutting up food? Opening a can? Fell?"

She shook her head.

"So what happened?"

I looked to her friends for an answer.

"I was trying to open a bottle of wine," she finally admitted.

"Okay," I replied. I knew she was underage, but I didn't think too much of it.

"Tell her what you were using to open it," one of her friends suggested.

The patient kept quiet.

"She was trying to get the cork out with a pocket knife," her friend told me.

"Ah," I said.

"But then my boyfriend texted me and I got distracted," the girl said.

"She almost ran us off the road," her fried added.

I rapidly turned my head in the girl's direction. "You were driving?"

She nodded. "Yeah. I kinda had a lot going on, huh?"

"You're lucky you didn't wreck. So let me get this right. You were texting and trying to open a bottle of wine with a knife while you were driving?"

"Yeah," she shrugged. "I've done worse."

I nodded. "Okay then."

I asked the patient if she had insurance with her and she sheepishly handed over her father's military identification.

"My parents aren't going to find out about this, are they?"

"Well," I replied, "I do have to mark it as a liability in my system because the accident didn't happen at home. It is possible someone from billing may be in touch with your father because he is the insurance holder, but I'm pretty sure details can't be discussed due to HIPAA."

"Oh, thank god," she sighed. "I was smoking pot and wrecked one night and the cop ratted me out."

Walk of Shame

We received word of a teenager en route via ambulance. The minor's diagnosis was listed as an overdose. Apparently, the teenager decided to smoke K2, which most people know to be synthetic marijuana and usually labeled 'Not for human consumption.' This decision resulted in the patient arriving in an unconscious state.

The patient's parents and his posse arrived around the same time. There were at least a dozen of the teenager's friends in the waiting room, with the patient's crush acting as the official leader of that group. The patient's mother wasn't having it.

"My son is grounded," the mother sternly explained to the patient's crush.

"But you haven't even seen him yet, have you?" the teenage girl sassed in reply.

For a minute, I thought the patient's mother was going to slap the girl for the attitude displayed. From the way she bit her lower lip and her left eyelid twitched, I'm sure she was considering it, too.

"I don't *have* to see him to know he's not going to be talking to *any* of his friends for a while," answered the patient's mother.

Defeated, the female teenager sulked back to

the waiting room and broke the news to the patient's friends. They didn't seem bothered by what the mother said, and they weren't leaving.

While the nurses and doctors in the back were getting the patient's vital signs and getting him settled, the patient's mother paced the empty lobby.

Finally, a nurse emerged from the double doors to the left of the registration desk and called the patient's mother to the patient's room.

I didn't go to the back to verify information because the patient's mother was in and out, in and out. She nervously walked in circles in front of the ER doors and smoked while she talked on the phone to the rest of her family.

Because the patient admitted to ingesting K2 but did not have the synthetic drug on his person, police could only interview him and remind him of the dangers of participating in drug usage. The patient was released to his parents four hours after he was initially registered.

The lobby was packed when I saw the patient's mother come through the double doors. The patient's friends were still in the waiting room, joking around while they waited for their friend. None of them dared to approach the patient and they all cautiously eyed the patient's mother, as if each and every young person in the waiting room feared the woman.

"Mom," nagged the patient, "this is so embarrassing."

All of the patient's friends were rolling in laughter, and several of the patients waiting to be registered snickered.

"You should have thought about that before you embarrassed me by making a bad decision with your life. Next time you think about doing something dumb, I want you to remember how you feel right now."

The patient continued through the lobby, wearing only a skid-marked pair of white boxer briefs and high-top sneakers. His mother held the patient's folded clothes in one hand.

Instead of leading the patient to the exit, the mother ordered her son to follow her to the waiting room. While standing in next-to-nothing, the patient was commanded to promise aloud he would never try drugs again, as well as explain in a brittle voice that he was grounded indefinitely.

Wacky Wednesday

It's not uncommon to see patients arrive at all hours of the day and night heavily intoxicated. We're generally okay with ETOH patients. Several arrive so inebriated that they don't do much else than sleep it all off. Every now and then we will encounter a belligerent drunken patient.

During the night in focus, not much was going on. From midnight to almost five in the morning, all was calm and we had only registered and treated two patients. It was so calm that I decided to take a break from filing patient information.

That was a mistake.

At 4:45, the charge nurse activated a 912 trauma for a patient delivered by ambulance. She had been involved in an MVA and required an immediate transfer to surgery.

While the nurses in the back were scrambling to prep that patient for the transfer, two EMTs escorted a young man through the double doors and held him from each elbow so that he could answer my questions and sign the consent form. The young man screamed that he was experiencing dental pain.

Each time I asked the patient a question, I had to repeat myself because he kept asking, "WHAT?!" With each question, the patient (and I) grew more impatient. After my fourth—and last—question, I explained to the patient that the triage nurse was escorting another patient to a room and would return shortly. The man seemed to accept this and went to the waiting room.

Just as this was taking place, two more patients arrived at the registration desk. Because I am the only registration employee on the overnight shift, I was beginning to wonder just how many more people would come in and I briefly felt overwhelmed the sudden influx in arrivals.

While I was registering the first new patient, I saw the man from the waiting room get up and walk towards the exit.

"Hey," I said to the EMT standing to the side of the registration desk, "is your guy leaving?"

He shrugged. "Hey, buddy," he called to the patient.

The man turned around.

"You can't keep people waiting like this," he shouted. "You can't expect them to wait forever. I have a real emergency."

Yes, it was such a *real* emergency that the patient, in the system (and waiting room) for a whopping three minutes, made the decision to leave the hospital on foot, in the rain.

(You know what we think when this happens? *'Well, at least I have one less patient to deal with. YES!'*)

As soon as I finished registering the patient in front of me, another took her place. I quickly registered her and sent both patients to the waiting room.

Just as I did this, a man wearing blue and white scrubs hurried through the front door. He was breathing unevenly and shaking.

"What's going on right now?" I asked, believing the patient was possibly experiencing a panic attack, strictly by looking at the expression on his face.

The man pointed to the parking lot.

"I was coming inside and there's a woman passed out in the parking lot. The girl with her asked if I could help get her inside, but I don't work here."

I interrupted him and called to the back to explain what the man had just said to me. Within seconds, three nurses ran to the lobby and left the building. Two more wheeled an empty hospital bed outside.

Not knowing if the unit clerk in back planned to register the parking lot patient or if I was expected to, I remained at the registration desk. The man at the desk was family for the MVA and was directed to the surgery waiting room.

A nurse ran back inside.

"I don't know how the hell we got so busy," she exclaimed as she sprinted to the back ER.

She was gone by the time I could shrug and she quickly ran back outside with a neck brace.

About a minute had passed before another nurse ran inside and asked the lingering EMTs to grab a patient mover from the ambulance. This would bring the count of staff members and emergency responders to the patient's rescue to eight. The patient was not responding to ammonia and she was still unconscious.

Finally, the patient was wheeled inside on a bed and was taken straight to a room. Her friend was sobbing and explained the two had visited a party and the patient went a little overboard.

A little overboard was an understatement. The patient's BAC was four times the legal limit. I hurried to the back to gather information from other patients when the drunk patient stopped breathing. The unit clerk called the operator and requested a stat page to Respiratory. While members of that department were en route, the charge nurse performed a sternum rub on the patient and then moved to using a pump respirator. Respiratory sent two staff members to the patient's room. Soon after their arrival, the patient began breathing on her own and came to.

"What are you doing to me?" she angrily demanded. "My chest hurts."

The charge nurse nodded. "You stopped breathing and were unresponsive."

Instead of, I don't know, thanking staff for

keeping her alive, the patient complained and badgered her nurses.

Back up front, I was able to speak to the patient's friend. As it would turn out, the patient was out drinking with her friends. When it became clear to the friends that the patient had consumed too much alcohol and needed medical assistance, they left her on the bathroom floor of a local pub. Instead of calling for help, the friends texted the woman in front of me. The woman then raced to the pub and asked bouncers to help transport the patient to her private vehicle. According to the woman at the desk, the patient's other 'friends' were more worried about getting in trouble for using fake IDs than they were about saving the patient's life. If the woman at the desk hadn't been there to transport the patient to the hospital, nurses stated the patient may have died.

In the end, the patient was discharged and didn't show much regret to her actions. In fact, she was laughing when she left and said she had a great time, despite passing out in the hospital parking lot and being admitted to the Emergency Room.

Worrywart

A new mother came in at three in the morning and registered her week-old baby. When I asked the mom what the problem seemed to be, she replied that the baby appeared generally healthy, but she was afraid the baby's nose was too big for, well, a baby.

Yeah.

Triage took the mother and baby for routine questioning before the patient was taken to a room in back.

Although doctors and nurses tried to assure the mother that the baby's nose was a 'normal' size, she insisted upon every type of test and exam possible.

She and the baby were discharged a while later.

Nothing was wrong with the baby. I can't say the same for the mom.

They Breed

Let me just say this: After working in the Emergency Room, I am convinced the opening scene of *Idiocracy* is taking place in reality every single day.

On a steady overnight shift, the hospital received a call over the radio that an ambulance was bringing in a 30-weeks-pregnant woman. The woman said she was bleeding and believed she was experiencing a loss of pregnancy.

When the woman arrived, I was surprised to see her diagnosis had been entered on the tracking board as: itchy.

"Itchy?" I asked the EMTs. "What happened to her thinking she was losing the baby?"

One of the first responders rolled her eyes and groaned. "I can't even talk about it. Go ask someone else."

I shrugged off the woman's response and gave the doctors and nurses a bit of time before I headed to the back to gather the patient's information.

"What's going on with this patient?" I questioned the unit clerk.

The woman laughed as I stood in front of her with a look of confusion on my face.

"She's something else," the clerk grinned.

"Okay," I sighed. "I definitely have to go find out what the fuss is about."

And so I did.

I knocked before entering the patient's room. She was lying on a half-reclined bed and she was fidgeting with her cell phone.

She smiled when I introduced myself, and I quickly ran through her information. I kept trying to think of a way to work in why she was there, but I was drawing a blank. Lucky for me, I didn't have to ask. She volunteered the information on her own when I mentioned, "Okay, since you didn't have an accident or injury, we can skip that screen."

"Nope," she stated. "I'm here because I'm itchy."

The patient then proceeded to tell me the whole story. See, she said her pubic area was itchy, so she scratched through her pubic hair for so long and with such force that she nicked her skin with her extra-long fingernails. In a short amount of time, the patient realized she was bleeding.

Now, this is where I have to break it down.

The patient noticed she was bleeding. But was the blood coming from her vagina?

No.

The spots of blood were coming from her groin area, directly underneath her pubic hair.

Well, when the patient saw this blood, she thought she had caused herself to go into labor.

Did she think the baby was going to pop out from her vagina?

Nope.

The patient thought the baby was going to tear through her groin area (yes, from the patch of pelvic space covered by pubic hair) and die because it was too soon for the baby's arrival.

I fought an urge to laugh and instead stared at the patient with a dumbfounded look on my face for what must have been a good 20 seconds before I finally blinked and silently nodded.

"Well," I quickly said, "I hope you get to feeling better. Try to have a better day."

The patient thanked me and I started to leave the room.

"Hey," she called to me. "A few of my friends are going to be here for support in case the baby comes, so can you send them to my room when I get there?"

I cleared my throat and nodded.

I parked my cart against a corridor wall and headed back to the unit clerk's area. I immediately laughed. In between my wheezes and snorts, I could catch conversations between nurses. They were all talking about the patient. One male nurse was reenacting the tear-through-the-flesh scene from *Alien*.

About 10 minutes later, a few of the patient's friends did arrive. Each and every one stated the patient sent a group text saying she was in premature labor.

The patient was discharged shortly after her friends arrived. Half of them left, cursing and muttering to themselves, before the patient received her discharge papers.

Reality

The first time I was in the ER when a patient died, it made me stop and think about how quickly life can change. A young woman, just out of her teens, had been seen in another non-trauma bay just two or three days earlier for ETOH. She stayed in the back until she came down from her high and then she talked to counselors for an hour or so. By the time I had gotten to the room, that patient was red-eyed and tired. She tearfully told me she wanted to beat addiction but wasn't sure how. Her parents arrived and took her home. The entire family seemed determined to get the woman's life back on the right track.

And then I saw her name in front of those dreaded words: Code 99. This code is similar to the Code Blue used in hospitals and thrown around in medical dramas on television. In layman's terms, it means the patient is dying and every available staff member capable of resuscitating the patient should get to that room *now*.

As I was staring at the tracking board, someone changed the Code 99 to DID, or 'died in department.' The patient's parents screamed and sobbed when they heard the news.

It was a surreal moment for everyone, I think. The patient was so young and never had the chance to *really* experience life. She had never been married, didn't have children, and she had never been to college. She battled her demons and lost.

Months later, when I was standing at the nurse's station just shy of an hour before my overnight shift ended, the charge nurse took a report of a self-inflicted gunshot wound coming in via ambulance. A male attempted suicide by shooting himself in the temple with a pistol he kept for home protection. According to the dispatcher, the man's wife was on her way to the hospital.

There was no hesitation in the room once the report was received. The charge nurse ordered one of the unit clerks to activate a trauma code. Every nurse in the ER that morning scrambled to find PPE gear and helped one another suit up in long-sleeved blue robes that tied in the back. With it being so close to shift change, there was only one doctor in the ER. Because the nurses were busy prepping a trauma room and both unit clerks were busy alerting other departments, the doctor took it upon himself to thumb through the directory and he began notifying surgeons on call.

The doctor stopped mid-conversation, almost as if he was halfway across the country when he remembered he left the stove on.

"Someone needs to discharge room eight before this guy comes through here."

The patient in room eight was four-years-old.

She was brought in by her parents because she presented vomiting and diarrhea. Her room was directly across the hall from the trauma room. I had just left that room and was fighting with the computer on my cart to wrap up her contact information. I knew there was no way to get out of that room without seeing the trauma room across the way.

Nobody spoke up. I'm not sure anyone actually heard the doctor.

"Hey," he shouted to anyone. "Get eight out of here now."

"Everyone's busy," one of the unit clerks responded as she ended her call to Respiratory. "Eight's nurse is prepping an IV."

The doctor shook his head and then handed the child's discharge packet to the unit clerk. "Hurry up and get them out of here. That kid doesn't need to see anything that's about to happen."

The unit clerk nodded and entered eight. As she did, I parked my cart against the corridor wall and restarted the computer. I would have to go back to the front to enter that patient's information, and then I could bring the face sheet back when I had an extra minute.

I started to walk back to the front but quickly dodged to the side of the corridor to make way for the EMTs running down the hall. Four first responders were feverishly trying to keep the patient alive. One used a pump respirator to force air into the man's lungs. Another checked the man's pulse.

"Mommy," I heard, "is that man hurt?"

I turned to see the child from eight gawking at the man on the stretcher. Her parents' mouths were hanging open and the girl's father glanced over to me. He didn't know what to tell her. We all saw the same thing. The adults in the room knew what the gaping hole in man's head and the blood dripping all over the place meant.

The girl's mother sniffled and said, "Yes, baby. That man is hurt."

"And they're going to make him better?"

The child's parents silently escorted her from the ER and I went back to the registration desk. All the way out the door, the little girl from eight kept repeating her question. Her parents didn't know what to say in response.

I hurriedly edited eight's information and printed a face sheet to the printer in back. As I was closing out of that patient's chart, a woman came through the front doors. Though she appeared calm and collected and couldn't *possibly* be involved with a suicide attempt, a pit in my stomach told me the woman was the newest patient's wife.

"My husband was just brought in," she told me. "He shot himself."

I nodded. "They just brought him in, so they're going to need some time to get him in the room and settled. Can you sign a consent form and answer a few questions for me?"

I knew the job still had to be done, but I couldn't help feeling guilty for knowing her husband was as good as dead, yet still going through his information casually.

"I think the bullet just grazed his face," she kept saying with a light smile. "He pulled the trigger and his hand jerked. So he'll be okay, don't you guys think?"

And then I knew I had to ask the question. In our department, we're supposed to ask each and every patient about a religious preference. It's not so much for religious beliefs regarding blood transfusions or prayer requests; trust me, if a patient believes that firmly in their faith, they won't hesitate to tell every nurse they meet. No. This question is one my coworkers and I ignore until something *bad* happens. This is the question we ask when everyone is pretty sure you're going to die.

"Does your husband have a religious preference?" I asked. The words slipped out from between my lips flawlessly, but there was a hard lump in my throat that wouldn't budge.

His wife nodded. I asked if she thought he would want his place of worship notified, to which she replied she thought he would.

I took a deep breath and said, "Okay, I'm going to let the doctor know you're here. Now, I hate that I have to do this, but I have to ask you to please wait on the bench in the lobby or in the waiting room. As soon as someone knows something, they'll be out to tell you. We understand this is a difficult time for you, so I know it won't be long before someone will come out."

The patient's wife was understanding and went to the waiting room. I rushed her husband's paperwork to the back. There were a few nurses in the room, but the doctor was walking away.

"Kerry," the nursing supervisor said to me, "the patient's parents were apparently notified by his wife."

"Okay," I said. "I'll let you know when they're here."

He scowled.

"Uh, no. You won't have to. Look, uh, after she got off the phone, I guess the patient's father had a heart attack. He's coming in as a Code 99. His wife said the entire family is on the way. I need you to do your best to keep the family calm and keep them out of here. Under no circumstances are there to be any visitors back here unless we come out and get them."

I nodded and went up front. Just as I was sitting down again, the doctor from the back went to the waiting room and asked the male patient's wife to come to the trauma room.

I watched the cameras. EMTs were hosing blood out of their ambulance and off the ambulance bay floor. Another ambulance pulled in and I knew it was the patient's father, accompanied by the first patient's mother.

Two paramedics rushed a stretcher inside while another wheeled in a panicking elderly woman. I could hear her shrieks all the way down the hall. Shortly after her husband's name showed up on the tracking board, hers did. She had passed out, fallen out of her wheelchair, and hit her head on the ground.

What a freaking mess.

Just when I thought it couldn't get any worse, the rest of the family rushed through the front doors.

"Take me to my parents and my brother now," ordered a man at the registration desk.

"Sir," I stated calmly, "I understand this is a stressful and scary situation, but the doctor is not allowing visitors right now. They're doing all they can do and are still in the early stages of trying to make everything better."

"I'm going back to their rooms," the man said again. His family cheered him on.

I picked up the phone to call security, but when they didn't answer, I was patched through to the operator.

"Page security," I requested in a hurry.

The operator replied, "They didn't tell you they were called to the back? They were supposed to tell you they couldn't be up there for a few minutes."

I hung up the phone and tried to remain firm, yet understanding.

"Sir," I said, "your brother's wife just went back. Right now, they're trying to stabilize your father and your mother has been admitted. Everyone we have is working as hard as possible, and when they know something, a doctor or nurse will come out to speak with you."

"No," the man shouted.

He attempted to pass on my right side, but I stood in his way and quickly shut the door to triage. Thinking back on it, he had me beat in size by a good 100 pounds and could have easily tossed me aside, but his family dragged him to the waiting room. For what seemed like an hour, I was surrounded by cries of fear and sadness from the waiting room and by shrieks of grief from the gunshot wound patient's mother from the back. I finally went to the back to see if I could get an update on anyone.

"Dad is going to be okay," the nursing supervisor told me in a hurry. "He's going up to Critical Care in a minute. Mom is still having some trouble dealing with everything. We're trying to get her calmed down, but we will probably have to administer a sedative."

"And the gunshot?"

He looked at me and knew I knew the answer, but I had to hear it.

"There's nothing we can do for him. He's showing only slight brain activity. His wife has agreed to donate his organs, but we can't do that until brain activity has completely come to a halt."

I glanced to the monitor displaying the registration desk and lobby. More family members were flooding in.

I nodded and said I had to go.

A tech came out and we tried to move some of the family to the consult room, but it just wasn't large enough. I directed the family to the chapel down the hall.

My relief walked in and stopped in his tracks as he saw the herd of people.

"What is going on right now?" he asked in a shaky voice.

I explained the situation, left work, and cried as soon as I pulled in my driveway.

People die. This, I know. There was a heavy sense of guilt weighing on my conscience. I couldn't forgive myself for knowing what was going on, yet going to the family and lying, pretending I had no information, pretending there was a chance that the bullet didn't cause the damage it did. I knew then and I know now that what I did was for the family's hope and faith and peace of mind, but I couldn't help but to think that when the first man's wife had flashbacks of that day, she would quite possibly relive standing at the registration desk and hearing my words of false hope on repeat. Would she know, later on, that I had lied the entire time? Would she feel bitter that she held on for too long to the belief that her husband had survived?

I went to work twelve hours later, still shaken by the events from that morning. It was still the talk of the Emergency Room. Nurses in the back were saying they were glad they didn't have to see everything unfold.

As I was clocking in, I learned the gunshot wound patient had been transferred to Critical Care. Several members of his family were at his bedside, knowing it was just a matter of time before he was declared brain dead. One nurse told me with a cringe that brain matter was leaking from the patient's head.

Security then alerted me of a situation at hand: a fight had broken out between the man's family, which resulted in a few members being arrested. Others were banned from visiting the floor.

When the patient's brain activity ended, his organs were harvested for transplant, and I think the man changed the lives of at least 10 other people. His parents survived.

Hours

The phone rang one busy evening and I answered.

"Emergency Room."

"Hi, yes. Can you tell me what your hours are?"

I hesitated. "Is this a serious call?"

"Uh, yes. I cut my arm pretty bad but I don't know if I can make it before you close. What are your hours?"

I explained to the caller that the Emergency Room was open 24 hours a day every day. He thanked me and we both hung up.

With a puzzled expression, I told my coworkers about the call.

"You should have told him we close in fifteen minutes and he needs to drive really fast if he plans on saving his arm," one laughed.

Order Me Around

I was alone on my overnight shift and all hell was breaking loose. My feet, calves, thighs...You know what? My entire body was sore from running to and from the back. Several patients lined up at the registration desk, making it impossible to offer privacy to fully gather information up front to take some of the pressure off, so I would register a handful of patients and then sprint to the back to drag my cart from room to room, praying the entire time that no newer patients were waiting up front.

For 20 minutes, I was in the back, gathering information.

"Patient up front," a unit clerk called to me.

I went back to the front to register the man, took a look around to make sure nobody else was lurking, and then I disappeared to the back again to hopefully gather information from the FOUR 911 traumas on the tracking board.

It didn't really surprise me that the rooms were filled with doctors and nurses, which meant I couldn't enter. I had been back there under five minutes when I stood at the nurse's station and separated my face sheets. One copy went to a plastic tray and would be handed off to the patient's nurse, while I kept the other copy for registration records. I glanced at the cameras between each paper. The lobby was empty. As I was separating the last set of face sheets, I looked up to see a patient in front of the registration desk. I hurried to the front and was nearly out of breath.

The woman at the desk wore an expression of irritation. She tapped her acrylic nails on the counter before she pushed the clipboard holding a signed consent form in my direction.

"Well," she spat, "it's about time."

"I'm sorry?" I asked.

"I've been waiting forever. I have an emergency."

"Ma'am, I'm sorry you had to wait. I've been looking at the cameras and ran up here as fast as I could."

"That's a lie," she said.

I ignored her. "Well, I'm sorry about your wait. What seems to be the problem tonight?"

"Other than having to wait in the *Emergency* Room?"

"I'm sorry, ma'am," I said, taking a deep breath. "I'm the only one here and—."

"Do you think I care if you're the only one here?" she shouted. "I have an emergency. I was supposed to get blood work done this morning, but I overslept and missed my appointment, so I need to get it done *now*. You know what? What's your name? I'm going to tell someone about you leaving the desk unattended."

I glanced at the clock. It was three in the morning.

"Ma'am," I said firmly, "we have four traumas in the back right now. I had to leave the desk to tend to emergency matters."

"*I'm* experiencing a trauma," she snapped. "I shouldn't have to wait twenty minutes to be seen."

It took great effort not to roll my eyes at her attitude or exaggeration, but I managed to restrain myself.

I registered the patient and handed her a stack of paperwork to give to the lab tech.

She didn't take it. Instead, she held up her index finger at me.

"Hold on," she said. "I have to go make a phone call."

The patient went outside and talked for 20 minutes before she came back in.

"Tell me how to get to the lab," she demanded.

I shook my head. "Sorry, but someone was hit by a car and since I was up front all of this time, they're being transferred with no information to give to the floor. I have to go tend to a *real* emergency right now. I'll try to find someone who's free and ask him or her to come up and give you directions so you can get the blood work done from the appointment you missed."

As far as I know, I was never reported. I don't think I would have cared much if I had been.

Friendly Reminder...

If you're prone to tripping and "accidentally" getting soda cans, candles, vibrators, or hairbrush handles stuck in your sexual orifices, you should probably keep these items off the floor.

"I'm going outside to smoke. Can you come get me when they call my name?"

—A patient with a complaint of 'shortness of breath' and 'coughing.'

I Cannot Tell a Lie

A male patient was brought in by an ambulance and had a diagnosis of: assault. For all assaults, nursing staff are required to notify the local police department. Most registration clerks here try to get in the room before the cops come because of the length it takes for the patient to be questioned.

During one overnight shift, I took my cart to one of the back trauma rooms. I knocked on the door frame before drawing the curtain.

The patient was in bed. One of his ankles was turned sideways and his pile of clothing to the left was splattered in blood. The patient's nose was crooked and both of his lips were swollen so much that he reminded me of a duck. One of his eyes were swollen shut and there was a bandage over a stab wound to his abdomen.

I gathered the patient's contact information.

"And now I have to do the accident or injury screen," I informed him.

"Okay," he croaked.

"Do you know where you were assaulted?" I asked.

"In an alley," he responded. "I was supposed to be running coke for this guy, but I took some of the package and did it at home. He found out and tracked me down."

"Wow," I stated.

"But you're not putting any of that on there, right?"

"I usually have to put exactly what the patient tells me," I replied.

He became frantic.

"But if you put that, my parents could find out. And my girlfriend will know that I do drugs. And if this guy thinks I went to the hospital and ratted him out, he's going to kill me."

"Let's just start over," I suggested. "What happened here?"

"I was walking home, minding my own business, and someone jumped out of a tree and started wailing on me. I didn't see them and they ran off without saying anything."

Two police officers arrived shortly after I left the room. When they were finished with the patient, one approached the desk.

"Did he give you the story about a homeless man attacking him?" the cop asked.

Her Life Story

I would estimate that a good 98% of patients love to talk about themselves. Sometimes it's hard to leave a room because a patient simply won't stop talking. It reminds me of talking on the phone with my grandmother. Though it could be 12:30 when she says she's getting off the phone, she quickly remembers something else to talk about, and the next thing I know is it's 3:00.

When I entered the room, I knew right away this female patient would be the same way.

"You look just like my daughter," she exclaimed. "The good daughter, though. The other two, they're just a mess. But you, you remind me of my good girl."

I swear, I think it took 10 minutes just to tell the patient I was from registration and needed to verify some of her information.

Another 10 minutes later, I had only managed to verify the woman's address and phone number. We were now stuck on the next of kin/emergency contact screen. The patient was going through every last one of her family members, giving pros and cons of why he or she would or would not make a good emergency contact.

"My grandson," she scowled, "stole a bunch of money from me last year. So there's no way I'm letting that little snot know anything. His dad isn't much better. I don't know how he turned out the way he did. I did everything I could to make sure he was raised right."

I nodded and tried to speak, but she continued talking.

After a great deal of encouragement, I persuaded the patient to keep her current contacts as her next of kin.

Next came the insurance screen.

When I asked the patient for her cards, she scrambled for her wallet and held out four items for me to grab. As I was separating the items, I noticed two were not insurance cards; they were family photographs.

"Oops," I said. I started to give the pictures back to the patient. "Don't need these."

She grabbed my wrist to keep me from returning to my cart.

"This," she said, motioning to the first person in the picture of 15 family members, "is my niece. She's dirty. She dances for money. She says she's getting married soon, but I think she's a dyke."

I gave an internal gasp.

The patient, indeed, wanted to point out each person in the photograph and tell me all about each one.

"This is my other son," she said. "He's really a good boy. I know I can depend on him. One time, I fell in the kitchen and couldn't get up. So I told my boy about it and he bought me one of those life buttons."

I nodded and forced a smile. I had been in the room nearly a half hour already. "That's nice."

She pointed to the woman next to her son. The woman in the photograph appeared nice enough.

"And that's one of my other daughters," the patient spat. "She's a dirty whore."

I was taken aback.

"Uh, okay."

"When she was still in high school," the patient said, "the principal called me and said my girl was performing sex at the back of the school bus for money."

I didn't know what to say.

"And she never grew out of it. She struts herself all over town. I swear, that girl's first baby came out walking and brought all of his luggage with him."

My eyes widened.

The patient leaned in and whispered to me, "That means she has a loose vagina, sweetheart. She got that way from all the men she's been with."

I nervously laughed. "Okay."

"Now, you don't go out and see all kinds of

men, do you?" she questioned.

"Uh, no. Look, I have to go, but—."

She interrupted, "Well, that's good. You don't want to have a loose vagina like my girl does. If she has one more baby, I think she'll be able to apply for a hotelier's license. That girl's got eight kids, I do believe."

"Okay," I announced, "I have to go, but—."

"If you're going to have babies," the patient said to me, "try to know who the father is, won't you? My daughter, she only knows one father. He's responsible for two of the kids. But he doesn't pay for them. We just know he's their daddy."

In a low-ball move, I asked the patient if she could dig through her wallet for her favorite picture of her kids. While she was doing that and talking to herself, I took my cart and left. I had been in the room for 35 minutes. Luckily, my coworkers caught other patients as nurses discharged them. I avoided nearing the woman's room at all costs and still feel guilty about it.

Mind=Blown

A teenager approached the desk with a woman I assumed was her older sister. Both young ladies were wearing bulky hoodies and tight leggings.

I asked the patient's name and date of birth. It turns out the younger girl was being seen for abdominal discomfort. She was 14.

And, I swear, the conversation was almost verbatim as the following:

"What seems to be the problem tonight?"

"My stomach hurts. It's more uncomfortable than it hurts, though."

See? Abdominal discomfort.

"And your sister is signing you in?"

The girl shook her head and looked at me funny.

"That's not my sister," she said. "That's my mom."

I almost fell out of my chair. When I scanned mom's driver's license, I took note that she was 27.

I sent the women to the waiting room. While they waited for triage to call, another woman joined them. I didn't want to make any further assumptions, so I simply made a mental note that another person had joined the women and left it at that.

Triage called the young lady's name and she followed the nurse to the triage room with her mother and the unknown other woman behind her.

"Do you have a shirt on underneath your sweatshirt?" the triage nurse asked the patient. "I'd like to get your blood pressure."

I glanced up and, in security's double mirror, saw the reflection of the patient pulling her sweatshirt over her head.

"Oh," the nurse exclaimed. "Are you pregnant?"

I whipped my head around to see the patient was carrying what looked to be a basketball under her tank top.

"Uh, yeah. I'm thirty weeks' tomorrow."

"Your paperwork didn't mention anything," said the triage nurse, looking over to me with a shocked expression.

"Well," the patient snottily replied, "I *did* tell her. It's not *my* fault she didn't tell someone."

"No, it is most certainly not. Do you have a local doctor?"

The patient shook her head.

"Okay, we'll have to see you in the ER. If the exam proves you need to go up to OB, it shouldn't be long until you get transferred, okay? And who are these two ladies?"

The triage nurse motioned to the second-oldest

woman first. "Is this your sister?"

"No," the girl snapped. "She's my mom. And this," she said of the other unknown woman, "is my grandma."

This time, I didn't *almost* fall out of my chair. I lost my footing and the chair rolled backwards. I stood, just as I felt my butt slipping from the cushion.

The triage nurse was momentarily stunned.

"Well," she finally announced, "you are just *the* youngest-looking grandmother I have *ever* seen, I tell you what!"

"I'm forty," the woman replied, clearly not amused or flattered.

I coughed on my soda and the patient and her family looked over to me.

"It went down the wrong pipe," I said with tears in my eyes.

I was doing math in my head. If I was right, the baby's great-grandma was 13 when she gave birth to grandma, and grandma was 13 when she gave birth to mom. Mom was doing slightly better than previous generations by waiting until she was 14 to give birth.

That's not the point of this story.

No, the point of the story is what happened when I entered the patient's room.

"Oops," I said, realizing there was a nurse in

the room, performing an ultrasound on the patient, "I'll come back a little later."

"You can stay," said the patient's mom. "Just get it over with so we can get out of here."

Hmmm.

I started to gather the patient's information, but I was distracted by the image of a fetus on the ultrasound machine's screen.

The baby kicked.

The patient shouted, "There. That doesn't feel good."

I looked to the patient's nurse. I'm pretty sure we had the same expressions on our faces.

"When he kicks?" the nurse asked. "That's when you feel discomfort?"

Let's keep in mind that the patient's nurse was 34-weeks-pregnant.

"Yes," the patient whined. "It's uncomfortable and I don't like it. Can you do something to make it stop?"

The baby lifted his arm in his mother's womb and jabbed her stomach wall.

"I don't like this feeling," said the patient. "It's really uncomfortable. I feel like this kid is just going to come tearing out of me, like in those scary movies."

The nurse bit her lips to keep from laughing.

"Sweetie," she said, "as the baby grows he has

less room to work with. My baby likes to lodge her head under my ribs. It doesn't feel great—sometimes it even hurts."

"I just want it to stop," the patient complained.

"Can't you give her some medicine to make it not hurt?" asked the patient's grandmother.

"I can't," the nurse answered. "I'm afraid this is just a natural part of pregnancy."

This answer upset the patient and her family. I quickly asked the rest of my questions and left.

Practicing

"What in the world are you doing?" the triage nurse asked an intoxicated, in-police-custody patient as he threw himself off the lobby bench and started flopping around on the floor.

"I'm having a seizure," he replied. "Help, I'm having a seizure."

"Get him up off the floor," the nurse told the man's arresting officer.

"But I'm having a seizure," the patient argued. "Why aren't you helping me?"

The triage nurse rolled her eyes. "Well, for one, people having seizures don't usually announce it while it's happening. Why in the world would you do that, sir?"

Defeated, he stood and swayed.

"Practicing," he said.

"For what?" the officer asked.

The patient smirked. "To get out of jail on medical leave, genius."

Shhh!

I was called to work early and walked in a mess. Someone had puked all over the lobby floor and two patients were "standing guard" until housekeeping could make it there. There were so many patients in the waiting room that there were no more empty chairs.

"Is it time to go home yet?" I joked.

My coworker laughed.

I looked to the tracking board. All but one patient was marked as completely registered. Unfortunately, that doesn't mean patients will be discharged; it just means registration clerks are finished gathering information and nurses are free to discharge patients when treatment is complete.

I asked where my other coworker was.

"She's in the ba—."

The man didn't get to finish.

"That woman is so rude," my second coworker growled. "She yells at me every single time I ask if I can come in, and this time she threw something at the door."

I glanced to the board again. "She's been here two hours already. And she won't let you in so you can finish registering her?"

Both coworkers answered in unison, "Nope."

"She's sent me away three times," my male coworker stated.

"And me four."

I shook my head. "What's going to happen is she's going to be discharged and the nurses are going to be jumping down our throats because we don't have her face sheet ready."

"I know," sighed the female registration clerk.

"Did she say why she doesn't want anyone in there? What's she here for?"

My male coworker chimed in, "She's here for a headache and leg pain."

"So she's dressed," I thought aloud.

"Unless she decided to get naked for a headache," replied my female coworker.

I thought for a second.

"I'm going to find out what's going on," I announced.

I went to the back and several nurses stopped me as I was setting up my cart.

"That patient's pretty grumpy," one nurse said to me. "Just a warning."

I rolled my eyes. "Yeah, okay. Thanks."

I dragged my cart to the patient's room and knocked on the door.

"Registration," I said.

"No," gruffly replied the female patient. "You need to go away. You're annoying."

I entered the room anyway.

"Ma'am, I'm sorry if you're feeling ill or in pain, but I'm going to get some information from you, and then I'll get out of your way."

"Get out of my room. The commercials are almost finished and my show will be back on."

"Ma'am," I reasoned, "if you don't answer these questions, your insurance won't be billed. Instead, the bill will go straight to the last address we have for you. What I'm trying to do is make sure you don't end up with an eight-thousand-dollar bill that your insurance won't cover because you were too busy watching your show."

The patient hissed at me.

I don't mean she scoffed and blew me off. No. I mean she turned her head in my direction and hissed like an angry alley cat.

"They turned off my cable at home and this is the season finale," she griped to me. "It's the reason I came here. I am *not* going to be interrupted or sent home and miss it. So get out."

That was it. The patient registered in the ER so she could watch TV.

Work it, Girlfriend

A female teenager was brought in at two in the morning by one of our regularly-visiting police officers. She was still crying and sniffling when she was standing at the registration desk.

"Medical clearance," the officer told me.

I couldn't help but to note the patient was wearing a hoodie decorated in printed marijuana leaves. I wondered what her exact charge was.

Once I registered the patient, the officer escorted the patient to a room in the back.

I soon went to the back to finish registering the patient.

When I was in her room, she was calm and didn't cry a single tear.

As soon as I left the girl's room, the officer went in to speak with her.

"But officer," she sobbed, "I'm just a good girl who made a bad decision."

I smiled at one of the nurses at the nurse's station.

"What a manipulative little..." I remarked.

The female nurse nodded.

"None of the guys believe she's doing what I said," the nurse told me.

"Oh," I laughed, "she totally is. She didn't cry at all while I was in there, but as soon as that guy got in there, waterfalls."

The nurse nodded and several of the male nurses gathered around us to listen to our conversation.

"She's just feeling guilty about her decision to drink underage," one of the male nurses rationalized. "She's emotional, so of course she's not going to cry in front of everyone."

"No," I said. "What she's doing is trying to cry in front of men because she thinks they'll find her cute and vulnerable. Trust me. Women know these things."

"No way," the male nurse argued.

"Wanna bet?" I asked.

And right there, just outside the patient's room, we started a betting pool.

"Watch," I said to the men.

I waited for the officer to leave and entered the patient's room.

"I just forgot the address you gave me," I lied.

She wasn't paying much attention to me. As she focused on the TV, she distractedly and calmly repeated her address.

"So I guess you got busted, huh?"

She grinned. "Again."

"Well," I said, "I hope your night gets better."

I left the room and the male nurses were rolling their eyes.

"That doesn't prove anything," one said.

"Go in there," I challenged him. "She's going to cry and two all-knowing women are going to split your money."

The male nurse scoffed and entered the patient's room.

Within 10 seconds, we could barely make out what the patient was saying through her cries.

It was an easy $5.

I Can't Believe You'd Say That

During our triage process, the nurse will ask a patient questions regarding his or her medical history, such as the following:

Have you had any surgeries?
Are you currently taking medication?
Have you experienced this ailment before?
When did this problem start? /How did this happen?

In addition to these questions, the triage nurse also asks if the patient smokes cigarettes, drinks alcohol, or does street drugs. If the patient responds 'yes' to any of these questions, the nurse then asks how much and how often.

We had an 'interesting' patient in triage. She was the type of person you could tell would be crazy before she opened her mouth.

"And it says here that the last time you were at the hospital you said you smoke two packs of cigarettes each day?" the nurse asked. "Is that still accurate?"

"Sure is," the patient answered loudly. She let

out an unfounded cackle that echoed down the hall.

"And do you drink alcohol?"

"Few beers a night."

"Okay. Now, are you still regularly doing meth, crack cocaine, and smoking marijuana occasionally?"

The patient jumped up from her chair.

"Why would you say that? Why would you even accuse me of doing those things? I mean, I smoke a little weed every now and then, but how could you even say that I do those other things?"

I thought to myself, 'Probably because of the way you're reacting right now.'

"Ma'am," the triage nurse said, "it shows you responded to these questions before and gave these answers. Do you remember answering these questions before?"

The patient began pacing.

"Man, I haven't done meth in two weeks. And crack...I haven't had crack in a day and a half. I can't believe you'd accuse me of that."

The patient was in because she wanted the doctor to write her a prescription for hydrocodone.

Mr. Smart Guy

The lobby was full, with some people touching shoulder to shoulder, waiting to be registered and sent to the waiting room with the other 50 patients waiting to be seen. I was not only waiting on the patient in front of me to sign the consent form and fish for her ID, but I was also working on a floor transfer, as well as taking information over the phone so I could transfer *another* patient as soon as I had a free second.

A man and his friend walked in. The man took one look at the line in the lobby, glanced at the full waiting room, and said to his friend, "Come on. Let's just go home and call an ambulance so we don't have to wait through all of this crap."

"Hold on," I said to the woman on the phone.

I stood and said loudly in reply to the man, "I'm telling you now: if you do that, every last nurse and patient in this ER will know and you will walk out of here the most hated person of the night. Not only that, but I will personally see to it that you spend some time in the waiting room while the EMTs and nurses are trying to find you a clean bed."

The patient turned red and waited to be seen.

He had an ingrown hair on his testicles.

Hanky Panky

A 16-year-old boy came to the registration desk at three in the morning, looking for his mother. The 41-year-old patient was brought in via ambulance for respiratory distress, back pain, and an ankle injury.

"She has someone else coming to see her soon," the son said.

I sent him back to the room to see his mother and went about my business on the decently-slow shift.

About 10 minutes later, another teenager showed up and asked for the patient by name. Assuming this gentleman was the woman's other son, I popped the double doors and allowed him to go back to the room. The first son emerged from the ER a few seconds later. He went outside to smoke.

Thinking I had a few minutes to run to the back and finish registering the patient, I entered her room.

"Well, I guess you're not her other son," I gulped.

The second gentleman from up front was not only lying in the patient's bed, but his hand was cupping her breast and his tongue was down her throat.

Yes. Yes, they were making out and fooling around in her bed...while she was a patient in the Emergency Room.

The patient pulled her hand out of the boy's pants and glared at me, angry that I broke up her tryst.

"I only have one son," she spat. "This is my boyfriend."

"Sorry," I said. "I really thought he was your other son."

"Why?" he demanded. "Because I'm only seventeen?"

"I, uh, didn't know you were seventeen," I replied. "But, uh...So, I'm here to get some information, and then I'll leave so you two can get back to doing, uh, whatever. Or maybe the doctor will come in and treat you."

"How long before he gives me pills?" asked the patient. "I've been in here an hour already."

I looked to the tracking board. The patient had been in the ER for 22 minutes.

"I'm not sure," I replied. "I really think it depends on your exam results."

"Well, I'm hurting in lots of places. I deserve medicine."

"I can tell your nurse to come in here when we're finished."

The boyfriend sat up and pointed his finger at me. "Hey. She's not answering any questions until she gets some Percocet or something."

I shrugged. "That's fine. I'll come back later."

I left the room and went back to the front.

Not long after that, our charge nurse escorted the patient's boyfriend out of the room. Apparently, the doctor had walked in and the patient had her legs spread for her boyfriend. The doctor restricted the boyfriend from the room.

You know, that young man honestly didn't seem to care all that much that he was kicked out of the old-enough-to-be-his-mother's room. He didn't seem to care that she tested positive for methamphetamine. Nothing about the visit to the ER seemed to bother him.

"Hey," he said to his girlfriend's son, "let's go back to your house and play some video games."

<u>Surely Not</u>

An ambulance driver (not a medic—this guy was from a private company) came to the registration desk in the middle of a crazy busy streak. The waiting room was filled by patients left waiting for at least three hours, and all the beds in the back were taken.

"Ugh," I moaned to the man. "Who'd you bring in now?"

He gave me a female's name.

As I printed a face sheet for him, I said, "Thank God. She's been here every single day this week. At least I know all her information is right."

"I can be good for something," he joked.

"Why's she here now, anyway?"

He rolled his eyes. "Well, I guess the cops found her sitting in the grass at her boyfriend's work. She said he was waiting for him to get a break, but she wasn't even at the right building."

"Well, don't bring anyone else," I joked.

"I don't want to. I've been up thirty-one straight hours because it's been so busy lately."

We said goodbye to one another.

The patient had been in and out during the rest of her visits, so I figured I'd go back to her room, confirm information and have her sign, and then she'd be released shortly after.

Yeah, no.

"Good luck," said the charge nurse to me as I approached the patient's room.

I groaned. "But she's been so good all these other nights."

"Well, not tonight."

Obviously. Tonight she was in the mental health room, a room with a thick glass door and curtain that could be drawn to protect the patient's privacy. In the room, in the corners of the ceiling, were video cameras that fed live stream to a monitor at the nurse's station.

I knocked on the patient's door and entered the room.

The second I walked in, I realized she was not in the same state of mind she'd been in all the other nights I had seen her.

For one, the patient was crying, but no tears fell.

"I'm sorry you have to be back in here," I said. "I just came to confirm that your information is the same."

"I'm not the same," she screamed at me in a strained whine. She lifted the bottom portion of her gown to expose bruised legs. "Look what your people did to me just now."

I tried to talk, but the patient continued.

"Look at this gash. They did this to me."

There was nothing where the patient was pointing.

"Well," I hesitated. "Can you sign for me?"

The patient *took off her gown* and was left topless and in a pair of flesh-colored granny panties that fit snugly on her sagging, wrinkled skin.

She rolled over with her breasts smooshed against her bed and she creaked her neck to look over her shoulder. She smacked the back of her upper thigh where there was a bruise half the length of my forearm.

"Look at it," she shouted. "Look at my spot. Look at all the injustice here."

"Ma'am," I said with a straight face, "I just need you to sign and then I'll go."

She rolled over and sat up. Her breasts reached down to the top of her navel.

The patient stretched out her arms toward me, with her forearms upward.

"I can't bear no more pain in my arms," she cried loudly.

"I'm guessing that means you're not going to sign..."

"It means I can't bear no more pain in these arms. Child, you're killing me. Do you feel good about it? Do you? You're killing me."

"Well," I announced quickly, "I'm going to go."

I left the room and threw my hands wildly in the air, the clipboard in my left hand jiggling in my palm.

"What the *hell* was that?" I asked loudly.

Several nurses watching the streaming feed cackled.

I went back to the front and continued with my crazy night.

An hour later, the patient was discharged. She was talking on her cell phone as she was walking through the lobby.

"They said the bottle started out with thirty pills. When I came in, there were only twelve left. I did *not* take all those other pills. Doing that would've left me a crazy mess."

"Which is exactly what she was back there," I whispered to my coworker.

The patient said, "Surely I didn't take all of those pills. There's just no way. All I did was snort some of [boyfriend's name] stash. That's all, I swear."

After a slew of tests confirmed their son was allergic to the new puppy waiting in their car, a couple left the ER and tossed the puppy out of the car. He wandered around the parking lot until one of my coworkers clocked out and took him home.

Ratting Himself Out

A shaking man wobbled to the registration desk and rested his head on the counter top.

"Can we help you?"

"I got tased. I need to see someone."

"Okay," my coworker responded. "Were you just messing around with it and got yourself on accident?"

The man shook his head. "No. The cops tased me but it didn't take me down, so I ran. But now I feel weird. I need to see a doctor."

We registered the man as a patient and he did see the doctor. He also saw the officers the nurses called while the patient was in his room.

Drink a Little Drink, Smoke a Little...It Had to Be Crack

We have seen our fair share of ETOH (drunk) and high patients. Here are a few stories:

* A college kid was wheeled inside by two police officers. He was so drunk he didn't know his name or birthday. And, since he didn't have an ID with him, cops didn't know them either. Nurses were insistent upon trying to get the proper information from the student so a next of kin could be notified. I thought I was making progress as the kid told me a month, but then he stopped talking and a blank look came across his face. He then leaned over and vomited. When I say he vomited, I mean the first spew was projected across the lobby and all the subsequent barfs created a pool that took up half the room. I popped the double doors for officers to take the kid to the back. He vomited down the entire hallway, leaving a trail of puke that reeked of sour alcohol. I called housekeeping and told them we had an emergency cleanup situation. I went to the back to give my John Doe paperwork to the unit clerk, but nobody was at the nurse's station. Every single nurse, tech, and doctor huddled around the patient in a trauma room. He continued to vomit and it sprayed everywhere. Nobody left the room with clean scrubs. Housekeeping spent more than two hours cleaning the lobby, the hallways leading to the back, and scrubbing the patient's room. He was admitted to Critical Care for the night.

* A drunk man came to the desk and said he had been bitten by radioactive spiders. He asked if he should have brought them with him, to which I wanted to laugh and nod, but I didn't because we were slammed and all the people behind the man were getting impatient. When I asked the man where he had been bitten, he disrobed in the lobby and proceeded to show me (and a shocked line of patients waiting to be seen) 'invisible' spider bites on his bare chest, abdomen, thighs, and groin area.

* A group of grown men decided to bring a charcoal grill inside during a February snowstorm so they could still 'grill out' and drink beer. They were too drunk to realize carbon monoxide was building up in the garage. The woman of the house came home to find the men passed out around the grill, with beer spilled everywhere. Nobody died, but one guy told me he wanted to as his wife continued to lecture him.

* One man was brought in by an officer for drug abuse (I guess the man was found in possession of crystal meth). The officer had to

give the man's name because the patient refused to say it. When the name was said, the patient flipped out and started screaming about how his parents were stupid and named him something equally idiotic. The name was something generic and 'normal' like 'Kyle,' but the patient thought his parents went 'overboard' and try to pick an 'artsy' name.

* Call that came over the radio in the back: unresponsive male, late teens, found passed out in a snow bank with an empty bottle of tequila. Treating subject for hypothermia and intoxication. The patient was brought in via ambulance and was transferred to Intermediate Care, but not before his mother showed up and started smacking her unconscious son with her pocketbook.

* Upon pulling in the full parking lot at work, I noticed eight squad cars parked in front of the ER entrance. I groaned and walked in the madhouse. Patients in the waiting were grew impatient and the back part of the ER was on lock down. The only patients allowed to leave were those being discharged. No new patients or visitors would be granted entrance unless the situation was critical. I went to the back. There were cops standing outside of six separate rooms. I asked what was going on. According to a frantic nurse, the patients were spending some time at a local

detention facility and were in on a scheme to manufacture drugs out of items they had access to during mandatory chores. Included in the drug mixture were splashes of the following: Comet powder cleaner, liquid dishwasher detergent, and ammonia. Each of the six patients ingested a large dose of the makeshift toxic 'drug' before they experienced seizures and fell into what were diagnosed as comas. Surprisingly, none of the patients died from ingesting the toxic mixture, though one patient coded twice in two hours. The last anyone at the hospital heard, the patients were facing sentence extensions for their risky behavior.

The Bottle Incident

It was a busy night and I was in the back, trying my best to keep up with the tracking board. As I was dragging my cart from room to room, I found myself walking toward a nurse escorting a patient and two friends to a room. The nurse sighed and rolled her eyes, and from the patient's attitude, I could see why.

"I told you," the patient snapped, "that I don't know who could've done it. Maybe if you'd listen you would know. One minute I was minding my own business, and the next thing I know someone smacked me in the back of the head with a glass bottle. And you know what? I have a cut on my scalp. There's glass in my hair. I shouldn't have had to sit in the waiting room for ten minutes. You should have gotten off your lazy ass and brought me straight back."

The patient was 19 and I was infuriated just at overhearing her as she walked down the hall. Yes. She walked. She was in such 'dire' condition that she walked. And *of course* she had been minding her own business. They all always are. If you're ever minding your own business, be on the lookout for 'some dude' or 'someone.' Seriously, this person is nuts, just going around and assaulting future patients.

I continued entering other rooms before finally giving up. Every room I tried to enter had a doctor or nurse inside, so I finally parked my cart along the wall, plugged it in to charge, and headed to the front. One of my coworkers took my place in the back, while another sat in front of a second computer at the registration desk.

We registered a few more patients. As I was registering an elderly woman with high blood pressure, the snippy patient I had passed in the back pushed in front of the patient at the desk and demanded immediate attention.

"Write me a note for school," she ordered me.

"I'm with a patient right now," I calmly responded, "and we don't write passes, anyway. Only the nurses in the back do that."

"Don't you tell me what you do," she shouted loudly. "They told me *you* write the passes, so you'd better start writing one now."

I repeated, "You'll have to talk to your nurse. If you can give me your name, I'll call her."

The patient looked at me with a glare.

"What's your name?" I asked.

Finally, after seconds of bitter silence, the patient tossed her wrist over the counter to show me her bracelet.

"You can't just tell me your name?" I asked, as I leaned in to read the bracelet.

"I shouldn't *have* to tell you my name. You

should *know* already."

"I didn't register you," I responded, reaching my level of tolerance.

"Did I say you did? Nobody goes through life and doesn't know me."

I scoffed and my coworker gasped.

I picked up the phone, and as I was dialing, I said to my coworker, "I swear to God, we've been so bu——."

The patient shrieked. "You swear? You swear? You're going to sit there like I'm not here and you're going to ignore me when I clearly told you to do something? This is unprofessional. Honey, *you* work for me, and you'd better start realizing it. I'm going to call in as soon as I get home and report you."

As I was waiting for the unit clerk to answer the phone—which I knew would take a while, anyway, since we ran out of clean beds in the back and there were five admits about to be transferred to critical care floors—I grabbed a piece of paper and wrote down my name. I then slapped it on the counter.

"If you're going to report me," I said, "make sure you spell my name right."

Of course, this action irritated the patient that much more. True, it wasn't the best action to take, and I've never blown up at a patient quite like that since, but I was at my wit's end.

The unit clerk finally answered.

"The girl in for a head injury is at the desk and she wants her nurse to write an excuse note for school."

"Oh," said the unit clerk, sounding surprised. "She's out there, with you?"

"I don't want the nurse to write the pass," the patient said. "You guys are so stupid."

She then walked over to the double-sided mirror to inspect her head before she checked her makeup.

"Yeah," I said to the clerk.

She didn't immediately say anything to me, but I heard her call out the name of the patient's nurse and say, "Your patient went out front."

The unit clerk then hung up on me.

"Well," the patient demanded, "are you going to do your job or not? Don't make me call someone down here to reprimand you right now, in front of all these people."

The elderly patient behind the girl was exceptionally quiet and patient. She only shook her head, which was what most other people were doing as they stood in line and watched the teenager go on her power trip.

The patient's nurse ran out of the triage room.

"Ugh," the patient said. "Finally."

"You need to come back with me," the nurse

stated angrily. "You haven't been discharged yet."

"And you," the patient snapped with her head bobbing all over the place, "said I didn't need stitches, which obviously makes you a bad nurse. I was *hit in the head with a bottle,* you dumb bitch. You can't just look at me and say there's just a scratch there."

The patient turned to me. "Write that note now. I have an eight-page paper due in seven hours and I haven't even started it. If I fail my class because you're too stupid to do what I've repeatedly told you to do," she threatened, "I'm going to make sure you and this entire hospital pays for it."

"If you don't like my *trained* medical advice," the patient's nurse stated, "at least come back here and finish paperwork. I'll write your note and you can leave."

"The sooner, the better," the patient spat.

"Yes," the nurse said, "I feel the same way."

The patient followed her nurse to the back and soon left the hospital with an excuse note in her left hand and a packet of discharge instructions in her right hand.

"I don't need this crap," screamed the patient. "You guys didn't help me, anyway. Someone comes in because they get hit in the head with a freakin' bottle and they get told they don't need stitches because there's just a tiny scratch? Sure, don't listen to the patient. Don't listen to the person who signs your pay check or pays your bills. Don't you idiots know I'm the one who's paying this bill? I go to school full-time and you're not even going to listen to me? I'm educated."

The patient tossed her discharge papers on the lobby floor. As soon as she walked outside, waiting patients started whispering loudly about the girl.

"You know what?" I asked my coworker. "I know it's probably wrong to say, but if I had to be around that girl all the time, I probably would have hit her in the head with a bottle, too."

What I've Learned from the ER

– The first few weeks (or even months) of working in the ER can be the worst you'll ever experience, and not just because of the patients and problems you see come through the doors. Many nurses openly admit to a sort of hazing they put new ER workers through. When I first started, I wanted to quit every single minute I was at work. If I asked for help I was ignored or openly mocked. If I made a mistake, no matter how insignificant, forget about having even six minutes of peace. As other new employees have come and gone, I began noticing the hazing from outside the circle, and I've come to a new understanding about the process. While the majority of the behavior was and still is grossly unprofessional, I cannot deny it made me a stronger employee and person. And, honestly, my coworkers and I are not just a team, but we are also a family. We have cried together. We become angry together. We help each other out when one's car breaks down or the weather is too nasty for someone living out in the boondocks. In the end, there's not much we won't do for one another. We have to be able to know we're each strong and trustworthy when dealing with life or death situations. Each shift is like a separate family. It takes time for everyone to get to know one another, but when we do, we're unstoppable and inseparable. Of course, there are certain aspects I dislike about my job, but despite the stress and the amount of complaining I may do about some patients, I care for them all on a human level and would go out of my way to help anyone. I can't name a single coworker who'd respond differently.

— Despite my previous advice to find a primary care physician and take all your stuffy noses and common cold symptoms to the office, I've learned there are exceptions because you can't always judge the severity of a patient's condition based on the surface complaint. Small children and the elderly should visit the ER after, of course, using common sense. It's not usually necessary to run to the Emergency Room just because your baby has a fever of 99.9. It's probably not helping you if you come in and say you haven't tried anything to bring the fever down. But I've seen babies come in with a fever and the underlying problem has been a serious life-threatening infection. I've seen elderly patients admitted for conditions I'd never imagine would lead to admittance, such as congestion or a bad headache.

— You should never take your chances when you're experiencing chest pain, but ask yourself a few questions before you come running to your local ER. Have you been coughing excessively or forcefully lately? Your chest muscles tighten and can lead to sternum pain that many people confuse with heart problems. That's another thing: have you had a heart problem before? If the answer is yes, come on over and see us. It's important to tell registration you have a heart condition or have had problems in the past. Other things responsible for false alarms are indigestion, excessive upper body exercise, and breast pain mistaken for heart pain.

– Sometimes you can't get through to people. We've seen many patients who have desperately needed to be admitted, whether as a full admit or simply under observation. But we can't really force anyone to stay. It makes us wonder why the patient came to the ER in the first place. Maybe it's denial. Maybe it's fear. I don't know. What I do know is that I've seen patients vomiting blood as they've walked back out the doors. I've seen people leave against medical advice, yet they come back two times the very next day, just to leave time and time again.

– I'm not at all against public assistance, but it's easy to see why so many people are bothered by it. Some patients abuse the system. Sometimes I think the patients think they have to use it just because they have it, but other times I try to think that they use it as a last option to being unable to find a physician willing to take public assistance as a payment. There are nights I still find it difficult to not find myself angry when someone presents a public assistance insurance card for something like getting pimples on her chin when she gets her period.

— It's better to be safe than sorry. A father once brought his child to the ER because the 1-year-old boy ate a pill the father accidentally dropped on the floor and could never find. The pill was a 1 milligram dose. When the father told me this, I internally scoffed and wondered why he was wasting his time and money on something that was unlikely to cause any damage. But after labs came back and exam results were in, the child was transferred to a pediatrics hospital due to his organs in the first stages of failure. If that father waited or thought the way I did, the child would have probably died.

— There is an incredible amount of job security in the ER, and I am reminded of that every single day, whether or not I'm working. I once watched my neighbor's teenager cross the empty street, run full speed, and try to hop over his brick-walled front porch. On the third attempt, he tripped and smacked his face on the side of the porch. That accident took the teen to the dentist, but it reminded me that people do stupid things *all the time*.

– I'm not superstitious, but it's true that all the crazy people come out when it's a full moon. It's also true that the second someone says or thinks it's not busy, all hell will break loose. I know this is the wrong section, but here's something we want to tell you: don't ask us if it's been busy, and don't comment on how dead it seems when you're there.

– We all know life is unfair, but the Gods of the Emergency Room remind us all of this repeatedly. Patients with diarrhea or those unable to stop vomiting sometimes have to sit in the waiting room for an hour. In bigger cities, people with knife wounds may sit in the waiting room for six hours. And then, as soon as it slows down, a patient with a broken fingernail comes in and waits four minutes. Two-year-old toddlers are brought in by ambulance because they stop breathing, or six-month-old babies come in because they were born with Congestive Heart Failure and are having another episode. God-fearing, at-church-every-service, donate-to-every-charity, feed-every-homeless-person patients come in for stomach pains and transfer to critical care floors because they discover they have cancer. Life is unfair. There are many instances when ER workers question everything. I don't have an answer to some of the things I see.

– People die. It's a truth we all know, but it doesn't get any easier when you've spent six minutes compressing someone's chest and being dragged away by a coworker because you can't accept that it's impossible to save everyone. Life is short. Life is not promised. A man walked in one night and said he had chest pain. He even joked with registration while he was waiting for a nurse to take him back. The man was young and didn't have a babysitter, so he brought his small son with him. Before the nurse could get the patient to a room, the man's heart stopped and he fell to the floor.

– It's not that I thought hospitals were clean places, but after working at one, I've walked out knowing these places are disgusting, even if not on the surface. There's no five second rule if you drop food on the floor here. You throw that food away, even if it's the only sandwich you have for your 12-hour shift. People come in and vomit, bleed, spit, and urinate on the floors. Bloody patients or those with worms in their stools seem to possess some unstoppable urge to touch *everything* possible, and there are times we can't get the place sanitized before the next patient steps up and starts touching everything, too. I've never seen the waiting room seats cleaned. That's not to say they haven't been, but after thousands of hours of work logged, I just haven't seen it happen. People come here because they're ill. Keep that in mind if you ever think these places are clean. They're not.

– Everyone should have an emergency contact at all times. If this isn't possible, keep a regularly-updated record of health someplace first responders will see it if they have to break in your house and pick you up off your floor. Have a friend or family member you can trust in case you're admitted and won't be home for a few days, or someone you can call if you need a ride after receiving a pain shot. So many people come to the ER alone and some of them can't go home to walk the dog. I've seen patients sit in the lobby for six hours as they wait out the time they have until their medication wears off and they can legally drive.

– For every secret I have, someone else has one that makes me think I'm doing okay. Patients come in after (or during) family fights. They come in with foreign objects inserted in their rectums or vaginas or noses or ears. There are times you just have to wonder *why* someone would stick a vacuum extension up their butt, but I guess the important thing to remember is that what's done is done and the only thing to do is move forward and look for a solution to get that ballpoint pen ink cartridge dislodged from an elderly patient's intestine.

– Working in this department is dangerous. It's easy to forget this because so many people are focused on fact that Emergency Rooms are where you go to get help. But registration clerks make first contact with all patients and if shooters come in, we're likely to be the first to die. Several employees enter rooms alone with violent or handsy patients. Some patients or family members don't take the final diagnosis or treatment plan very well. It's scary to have someone throw something at you or wonder if that disgruntled patient is lurking in the parking lot, waiting for you to come outside.

– After entering the rooms of drunks, guys whacked out on bath salts, and a half-naked 400-pound man in the ER for experiencing chest pain and getting asked out, I've come to the conclusion that men have no shame.

Friendly Reminder...

If you like going through life with five fingers on each hand, remember it's generally not a good idea to use power tools and alcohol at the same time.

A Handle on Things

A tall, dark, and overall-attractive man approached the registration desk with tears in his eyes.

It was obvious he needed help, so I asked his name and date of birth.

When I searched for the man's name, nothing came up.

"Have you been here before?"

He shook his head.

"I need to see a photo ID and I'll take your insurance card if you have it."

He hesitated.

"Is there a problem?"

He finally sighed and reached for his wallet. "I just gave you a fake name."

"Ooookay," I replied. "Let's start over with your real name."

I entered the patient's information and we started over.

"What's the problem tonight?"

The man looked away.

"Sir," I said, "we've seen it all."

"You haven't seen this," he mumbled.

"You don't know that. Ballpark it for me so the nurses know which room to put you in."

He looked back to me and leaned in. When he spoke, it was such a soft whisper that I couldn't hear him.

"I didn't quite catch that," I said.

He looked to both sides and behind him. He stretched his neck to make sure I was the only person behind the desk.

He coughed, "I'm bleeding."

"Penile or rectal?" I asked without blinking.

He fidgeted. "The second."

"Okay, just sign the top line of that consent form, and we'll get you back to triage."

He was shifting his weight. "Uh, how long do I have to wait?"

"It shouldn't be too long at all. Maybe five or so minutes."

"There's a lot of blood."

"Are you bleeding through clothing right now?"

He shrugged and leaned in again. "I put one of my wife's pads in my underwear, but it feels all mushy. I can feel it just oozing out."

"I'll call the back and let someone know."

"Does everyone have to know?" he cringed.

I shook my head. "We take privacy seriously here. But I have to let the charge nurse know so she can assign you a nurse and the proper room."

He nodded.

"You're not going to ask me to sit down, are you?" he worriedly questioned. "Because I can't. I already feel like I'm wearing a diaper. I can't sit."

"You don't have to. Hold on just one second and I'll call the back."

The man paced around the lobby and I called the charge nurse to explain the situation.

"I'm sending someone right now," she said.

His nurse was a cute redhead with a button nose. Oh, and she was brand new to the ER after transferring from the pediatric floor two days earlier. And during her two 12-hour ER shifts, she primarily handled congestion and runny noses. She didn't seem nervous.

But the patient had taken to cracking every joint he could.

"Is, uh, there anyone else?" he asked. "Maybe I can, uh, find someone who's not as..."

The man chuckled nervously and gushed to the nurse, "You're really pretty and this is so embarrassing."

"I'm really married, too," the nurse joked. She pointed to his ring finger. "Looks like you're married?"

He nodded.

She shrugged. "We're professionals here, and

there's nothing to be embarrassed about. There's not much we haven't seen."

The patient reluctantly followed the nurse back to a non-trauma room. Within 10 minutes, the charge nurse called to the front to notify me of what I already noticed on the Tracking Board: the patient had been transferred to a trauma room.

I minded my own business until the nurse called again.

"I need you to get his information," she said. "He's going to surgery and his family's out of town, so nobody's going to be coming in for him."

I quickly headed to the back and grabbed my cart. Any nurse not in the patient's curtained-off room was standing in a circle, whispering to all the other nurses there.

"What's happening right now?" I asked one of them.

"He has a perforation."

"From what?"

The nurse started to explain but couldn't finish through laughter.

I waved her off and went to the patient's room.

When I opened the curtain, the patient was face-down on his bed and his bare butt was in the air. Two nurses and both doctors from the shift were standing over his buttocks.

I widened my eyes, as if to ask one of the

doctors what happened.

The patient was calm, right up to the point when I asked him if he had a living will or power of attorney.

"Oh my god," he screeched. "Am I going to die from this?"

"It's unlikely that you're going to die," one of the doctors stated firmly. "But we have to get you moved to surgery immediately because you're losing an incredible amount of blood and there is no way for us to stop the bleeding."

"If you help me, God," the patient bargained through his sobs, "I'll never do this again. Like, ever."

I left the room to allow the doctors and nurses more time with the patient. Then I head straight back to the circle of whispering nurses.

"Okay," I demanded. "Someone has to tell me what that was all about."

"He was constipated," the charge nurse explained, "so he inserted a fork handle to try to ease out the bowel movement."

"And jabbed himself?"

"Yes," she nodded. "He said he sneezed and the handle slipped."

The man was taken to surgery. Nobody mentioned him again, so I am assuming he didn't die.

Helpful Hint:

Take your shirt off *before* you iron it if you don't want to end up explaining how you sustained second-degree burns on your chest.

The Best Kind of Friend to Have

A 20-something-year old patient was brought in via ambulance for an overdose. According to the patient's husband, he and his children returned to their home to find the patient unconscious and surrounded by cocaine and prescription barbiturates – none of which were prescribed to the patient, but to some of her friends. It was obvious to the husband that his wife had her friends over to do drugs, judging by multiple cups of alcohol strewn around the living room, music blaring, and that the home was left in general disarray. Police officers theorized the patient and her friends were doing drugs and when she passed out, her friends panicked and bolted.

Shortly after arriving to the ER, it was agreed the patient should be transferred to ICU.

For the first night, the only visitors to and from the patient's room were her husband, two young children, and a few members of her immediate family. She was cleared from the ICU the next morning and was transferred to a general med floor, where she was in stable condition. Apparently the patient had come to, but she was not speaking much. She refused to explain what happened.

During her time on the general med floor, the patient received another visitor: a rail-thin female with sunken eyes and cheekbones. The woman's skinny jeans were hanging loosely from her anorexic-looking frame.

The patient was fine during and after the first visit.

The second visit wasn't so great for the patient. After the visitor left, the patient coded and was transferred back to the ICU, where she was stabilized. She remained unconscious for several days.

When she came to again, her husband demanded to know what had occurred in their home and why she would make the decisions she did when she had a family. The husband became so upset security was called and he was escorted from the floor until he could regain composure. Before the husband left, he was screaming that the family did not have insurance. The hospital bill for his wife was already over $40,000.

Meanwhile, the patient's friend showed up and was given a visitor's pass to the floor. Again, after she left the patient's room, the patient coded and was unconscious.

It was determined the 'friend' had been slipping the patient more drugs during visits. The last dose was the approximate dosage the patient ingested when she was first brought to the hospital just a week before.

In the end, the friend was arrested. Unfortunately, the patient never regained consciousness and died two days later. Her husband and children were inconsolable and spent hours in the hospital's chapel with counselors and chaplains before they were able to go home and start over again.

Whoops!

At the tail end of a non-stop, hold-your-pee-for-eight-hours-and-try-not-to-pass-out-from-low-blood-sugar shift, a male approached the desk in a wobble. His hands were trembling and his eyelids were twitching.

"Do you need to be seen?" I asked.

The patient opened his mouth to speak, but no words came out at first. I remained patient and waited for the man to speak. When he did, his words were strung together as nothing more but unintelligible gibberish.

"Sir," I asked, "can you try speaking for me one more time?"

He tried to talk again, but out came the same gibberish.

I recognized the man's symptoms as signs of a stroke, so I immediately picked up the phone and called the charge nurse.

"Chest pain?" she sighed. It would only make 12 that night.

"I think this man's having a stroke," I replied.

"Tell me what's happening right now."

"Hold on," I said.

I looked to the man. "Sir, can you please smile for me?"

The man curled his lips in a tight closed-mouthed smile. Just as I suspected would occur, one side of his mouth lifted upward, but the other half remained droopy.

"Only half of his mouth went up," I said in a hurry to the head nurse. "I need someone up here."

The rest was a blur. Three nurses came running through triage and the patient back there (and the triage nurse) stood up and peeked through the open doorway to see what the commotion was about. I sat down and let the professionals take over.

"Sir, can you tell us your name?" one of the RNs asked.

Again, the patient responded in a jumbled mess.

In response, the nurses urged the patient to take a seat in a staxi wheelchair and they took him straight back to a trauma room—the only room available.

As soon as the patient went back, I looked over to the tracking board to see a patient was being discharged.

"Hey," I told my coworker, "I'm going to the back."

When I went to the back, the scene was chaotic. Nurses were running to and from the stroke victim's room. All three of the doctors on the evening shift were yelling information to the two doctors coming on for the overnight shift. Two unit clerks were in the patient's room, each hoping to somehow catch the patient's name and date of birth. Most of the other rooms were considered to be on hold while everyone tried to figure out the newest patient.

In this industry, it's not rude to go about your business. Unfortunately, we are all too well aware that the world doesn't stop spinning during every crisis. There is always a job to do, and I had to do mine.

So, like usual, I rolled my cart to the room of the patient being discharged and I asked my normal questions. Nearly all of the patient's information had changed, so it took about a total of five minutes before I finished.

As soon as I rolled my cart out of the patient's room, the charge nurse wiggled her index finger hurriedly at me.

I rushed over to her.

"What's wrong?" I asked.

"Something very bad has happened here," she frowned. "And we're all going to need your help."

I was puzzled. "What happened? Oh my God," I gasped. "Did that stroke guy die?"

She shook her head.

"He wasn't having a stroke," she said. "His wife is the person we just discharged."

I looked back to the room I just left and then back to the charge nurse.

"No frickin' way," I blurted out. "That man *had* to have been having a stroke. He couldn't talk. He couldn't smile."

"He has a disease that affects his nervous system," the charge nurse told me. "He was only here to pick up his wife."

The nurse then explained how everyone agreed the man was having a stroke, but one of the techs in the room recognized the patient as one from years before. Apparently, the patient had spent some time in rehab where the tech previously worked.

"We all have to notify the Nursing Supervisor," the nurse informed me.

"Are we going to get in trouble over this?" I panicked. "I really can't lose my job."

She bit her lip. "We have to report it and document everything that happened. It's important if the family decides on litigation."

The 'stroke victim' was released as soon as the tech recognized him and he met with the Nursing Supervisor on call. He and his wife were incredibly understanding of the situation and the man actually *thanked* the ER staff for acting so quickly to remedy the situation that wasn't actually happening.

Friendly Reminder...

While I will <u>never</u> encourage someone to commit suicide, it is important to consider what you will do or become if your attempt fails. A gun to the head, noose to the neck, or running full speed at a wall with a knife's tip at your chest does not always work the way you planned. Outcome possibilities include permanent brain damage, paralysis, mental health evaluations, meetings with family and friends to explain your reasoning, hundreds of thousands of dollars in medical bills, and arrest.

Seriously?

    Please, **please**, <u>***PLEASE***</u> come to the ER at 4 a.m. because your anti-psychotic medication is causing you to experience erectile dysfunction. Yes, we know you 'only decided to come to the ER because [your] wife is *so mad* at you for *not being able to climax after an hour and a half.* Thanks for explaining that *after* you've asked three staff members to have sex with you.

<u>No Chance</u>

A college student registered with a diagnosis of 'vaginal bleeding' after explaining to me that she had a pregnancy termination the month before. She didn't have to wait to be seen. The triage nurse was hanging out in the empty waiting room, watching TV, and took the patient straight to the triage room after I signed her in.

The patient explained her situation to the triage nurse.

"So you had a pregnancy termination last month?" the nurse asked. "Do you think your bleeding could be your period?"

"No," the patient huffed. "It's not enough blood to be my period."

"So it's more like spotting?"

"Yeah, I guess."

"Is there any chance you could be pregnant?"

"No," the patient stated.

"Are you currently sexually active?"

The patient answered, "Yes. A few times a week."

"Do you use birth control?"

"No."

"So there *is* a chance you could be pregnant?"

The patient argued, "No."

"If you're sexually active and aren't using birth control," the triage nurse calmly asked, "can you please explain to me how it is that there's no chance you're pregnant?"

"Well, because I don't want to be."

I snickered.

The triage nurse fell silent for a moment.

"Ooookay," she finally said to the patient, "let's get you back to an exam room."

It didn't take long for a female doctor to perform a pelvic examination on the patient and to order two pregnancy tests—one testing urine and the other testing blood.

I heard the patient scream a slew of obscenities from the back.

"So," I asked the triage nurse, "what's that all about?"

I was sure I had a pretty good idea already.

"She's pregnant."

I guess there was a chance after all.

Helpful Hint:

If we tell you to sit in a wheelchair, stop arguing and just do it. I can't lift 300 pounds off the floor, and it's a lot quicker to get you to the back if we don't have to get a crew of lifters to the lobby in the middle of a busy shift.

A Long Way Down

A patient was brought in by her neighbor. The young woman was sobbing and clutching her right leg.

"Help me," she cried. "Help me."

"What happened here?" I asked.

"I think it's broken."

The patient's leg *was* broken. What caught my attention, though, was her story.

According to the embarrassed patient, her boyfriend dumped her earlier that day. After feeling that her life was over and she'd never find happiness again, the patient decided to commit suicide.

So the patient went to the second floor of her two-story home and opened a window. She said she took a deep breath before taking the leap. Honestly, she thought the 18-foot fall would end it all, but she landed feet-first. She realized she couldn't walk, so she screamed for help. Her neighbor came outside and brought her to the Emergency Room for treatment.

A mental health counselor talked to the woman and concluded the girl was not truly suicidal, but just not thinking clearly after the breakup. The patient left with a cast and a prescription for pain pills.

Won't be Shaking Hands for a While

It's not unusual for people in this area to see Amish community members traveling through town via horse and buggy. Some of the community's members even have driver's licenses to help out their families and friends in time of need.

Every now and then, the ER sees an Amish patient. Quite honestly, from my experience, if an Amish patient registers, I already know the patient is going to be made a full admit to another floor or will be transferred to another hospital—if he or she does not sign out AMA after receiving an exam. These people seem to have a better grip on handling medical situations than anyone else I know, and if they *have* to come to the ER, it's like they already have a general idea that it must be *really* bad.

Examples of this include the following:

* A mother and father brought in their small daughter after her sister threw a softball and it smacked the girl in the back of the head. The girl seemed fine, absolutely fine. Her pupils weren't dilated. She wasn't dizzy or confused. The child was jovial and energetic. Directly after her CT scan, though, the patient was transferred to a children's hospital in Columbus after being diagnosed with an intracranial hematoma.

* One man was brought in by ambulance with what EMTs believed to be a broken neck. The patient had been at the top of a 50-foot ladder, painting a barn, when he became dizzy, lost his foot, and plummeted to the ground. After multiple scans were done, doctors discovered the patient had sustained an injury in which he was internally decapitated. He was stabilized and flown out.

In other cases, doctors have diagnosed Amish patients, but the patients decide the injuries or illnesses are just 'bad enough' to need to visit the ER, but not 'bad enough' to be admitted.

With this patient, the circumstances were just a little different.

See, this Amish patient was from a different community in Pennsylvania. Unlike the local Amish, who live with electricity and modern technology to some extent, the patient's community did not. The two communities were brought together by a marriage, and the patient was in town to attend the wedding. Because there were no more beds to share within the Amish community, some of the travelers stayed in local hotels.

Well, this patient had seen electricity before in form of overhead lighting or television, but he apparently didn't have any experience with microwaves. One morning, he decided to pop his mug of coffee in the microwave for a few extra minutes while he took a quick shower.

As the man was about to get in the shower, he heard a small explosion and smelled smoke. He ran to the breakfast nook area of his hotel room to find the microwave had caught fire and the flames were spreading to the room's curtains. The man panicked and tried to extinguish the flames by swatting at them—with bare hands.

The man sustained second and third degree burns to both palms and could not move his fingers. The man was transferred to a burn unit a few hours away.

The culprit of the fire was the mug. It wasn't porcelain. It was tin.

Triage Nurse: "Have you been out of the United States in the last six months?"

Patient: "Yes."

Triage Nurse: "Okay, can you tell me where you traveled?"

Patient: "Well, we had to go to New Mexico for my wife's aunt's funeral."

Geography is hard.

<u>Drugs are Bad</u>

A little after two in the morning, two females walked through the front doors. One woman, younger and frazzled, was talking on a cell phone.

"Look," she said to me, "I don't really know this woman. I can't even tell you her name. I just know she obviously needs some help."

"She's a liar," the other woman yelled to me. This woman was in her late 40s and was struggling to carry in six bags of luggage. "She kidnapped me and punched me in the side of the head."

The woman was speaking quickly and her breathing was rapid.

"No," the younger woman said. "Look, she asked me to call her ex. He's on the phone now. Can I give you his number, and can I get the hospital's number? I'd like to get you guys connected so I don't have anything to do with this anymore."

The older woman continued to pace around the lobby. She dropped all her luggage and wildly kept trying to tell me her side of the story.

She leaned over the counter and whispered loudly, even though the other woman was right in front of me, writing down the other woman's ex's phone number.

"This woman kidnapped me. I need to see a doctor. And I need you to call the police. She hit me in the head. My whole body hurts. They have my cell phone and won't give it back."

"Your phone is in my car," the younger woman snapped. "If you want it, go get it now. When I leave, I'm not coming back."

"I'm not going back to your car. You're just going to kidnap me again and my stuff will be left here at the hospital and they won't give it back."

I sighed. "Ma'am, let's get you checked in. Do you still want to be seen by a doctor?"

She nodded several times. "Well, yes. I told you, I need to see a doctor because this woman hit me."

I looked to the younger woman. She handed me a phone number and I gave her a business card with the hospital's phone number.

I looked back to the patient and asked for her name and date of birth. While I was registering her, the younger woman left.

The patient started freaking out even more. I put her diagnosis as 'mental health' and finished her registration at the front desk so I wouldn't have to go to the back and see her again.

By the end of her registration, the patient was yelling and sweating.

I started getting nervous and knew both security guards were off in another part of the hospital, so I called the triage nurse.

"Hello?" she answered.

"I need you up here right now," I whispered to her.

"On my way."

I had encountered many other mental health patients before this woman, but she was so talkative and upbeat one minute, but threatening the next that I couldn't anticipate what was coming next. One second she'd be as sweet as could be, but the next she would lean over the counter and scream at me. I really started to feel that my safety was at stake.

The triage nurse came up in the middle of the patient's screaming and called the woman's name according to the paperwork.

The patient changed her tone quick and started crying. "You're not the police."

"Uh, no," the triage nurse said. "I'm here to triage you so we can take you back to a room for medical treatment."

"I never said I wanted medical treatment."

The patient started *spinning in circles.*

I looked to the triage nurse and growled. "Yes, she did," I whispered. "I swear."

She nodded.

Then the patient stopped spinning and swayed from dizziness. She was still crying. "I just need the cops. Go back there and get one out here."

"Ma'am," the triage nurse asked, "you are aware that you're in the Emergency Room, right?"

"YES!" the patient sobbed. "But my rights have been raped and I need the police. Go to the back and get the police, now."

While the triage nurse worked to calm the patient, the charge nurse walked to the front and stood in the triage room. She motioned to me and I walked over to her.

"What the hell is going on?" she asked.

"This woman is nuts."

"Is she being seen?"

I shrugged. "First she said she wanted to, but now she's saying she never said that. She's saying she wants the cops now, but she seems to think we have a few hiding in the back. I don't know if she's high or just crazy or what. Triage is trying to get her seen, I think."

The patient noticed the charge nurse and rushed to the woman. "Oh, are you the police?"

Our head nurse looked to her scrubs and back to the patient with a smirk. "Uh, I'm the charge nurse of this Emergency Room tonight. What's going on out here? Do you need help?"

The patient nodded. "I've been kidnapped and dropped off here. I need to talk to someone and I need the cops called. Can you do that for me, sweetie? You look like such a nice girl."

"Well, we can do that. Do you want to come back here to be seen while we're calling them?"

This is when the patient flipped out again. She started cursing and kicking her luggage around the lobby. While the triage nurse worked to calm the patient again, I called the operator to stat page security, and the charge nurse disappeared to the back.

Within minutes, both security guards were at the ER registration desk. The patient was pacing between the lobby and the waiting room. Our head nurse called up to the front to let me know the police were on the way. Security had their hands tied. Each time they would ask the patient to leave, she would say she wanted to be seen by a doctor. We couldn't refuse the patient medical treatment. But when it came time for the patient to come to the back, she refused to do that.

Security decided it would be best for the city police to handle the situation.

When the cops arrived, the woman took almost a half hour telling just part of her story. According to the patient, she was living with the woman responsible for bringing her in. The woman and her boyfriend allegedly woke the patient by punching her in the temple and told her they were all going on a drive to Wal Mart. The patient said she didn't want to go, but the other woman and the man forced the patient to go by holding a knife to a throat. The patient never said how her luggage got packed or ended up in the car.

According to the patient, on the way to Wal Mart, the three stopped at a gas station. The couple allegedly turned on the child locks so the patient could not get out the back doors of the vehicle, leaving the patient stuck inside.

One of the officers said what we were all thinking: "Ma'am, are you aware that you sound and act as if you are tweaking?"

The woman started to sob again. "I am the victim here. I am the victim. I want justice. I want those people arrested for what they did to me."

"But you can't tell us their names," the officer stated.

"No, I can't," the patient yelled, "because they gave me fake names that I can't remember, but God told me they were fake names."

"And you can't tell me where you were living."

"Because they blindfolded me."

The patient had an answer for everything.

"Okay," the officer sighed. "Look. You have a few options right now. First, you can be seen by a doctor and have your mental health evaluated. Second, you can admit that you may have a substance abuse problem and we can try to get you a room at rehab facility. Or, if you don't want to do either of those, you can leave here peacefully or you can refuse to leave and go to jail."

The patient screamed at the officer and pulled at her own hair. "I am a victim. And you're telling me I'm tweaking?"

"Ma'am," the officer said, "you are surrounded by professionals trained to recognize the signs of drug usage and you are fitting the profile like a poster child. Now, we can call your ex-husband. Would you like us to do that?"

It was like the stars aligned or something, I swear, because just then my phone rang and I answered.

"My ex-wife is there," a male caller explained, "and I just want you to know I am not picking her up because she's psychotic. I kicked her out last week."

I interrupted the patient. "The police are here. Would you like to speak to one of the officers?"

Instead, the triage nurse took the phone. I had to go to switchboard to relieve the overnight operator for her break (because everyone in the hospital gets one except ER registration), so I missed the phone conversation between the patient's ex and the nurse.

"Sounds like you guys are having fun down there," the operator said to me.

I rolled my eyes.

"There's a crazy lady down there. Cops are saying she's on drugs. She won't leave or be seen."

When I went back to the ER, I expected the situation to be remedied.

But we couldn't be so lucky.

The patient was now sitting in the back office, directly behind the registration desk, and she was crying as she spoke on the phone.

"I was your wife for ten years," she sobbed. "And you kicked me out because I broke a few windows? What kind of good husband does that? Huh? What kind of good husband does that? Not a good one, that's for sure."

I groaned and asked the cops, "Is she going to stay here all night?"

One officer shrugged. "We're trying to get her out of here, but we'd prefer she not be walking the streets and bothering other people."

The patient got off the phone.

"Well," the officer asked her, "is someone coming to get you?"

She shook her head. "No. He said he doesn't want anything to do with me."

"He told me he'd be willing to work on your relationship if you would be willing to get some help for your addiction," the triage nurse said. "Now, we can get this process started, if you'd like. We have a lot of patients here for detox. There's no shame in getting help. It's actually a very admirable thing to do, to admit you may have a substance abuse problem."

"I don't have a problem. You have the problem. You're the one working in the middle of the night."

Good comeback.

The patient appeared to have a bright idea. She looked to the officers and asked excitedly, "Do you know the sheriff?"

One of the officers nodded but looked confused. "I do."

"Well, so do I. And I know his wife. She makes dresses. And they're just beautiful. She charges an arm and a leg for them and would sell more if she—."

"Ma'am," the other officer interrupted.

"Anyway," the patient digressed, "they'll take me in. I just know they will. Let's call them."

"I am *not* calling the sheriff at three in the morning," the officer stated firmly.

"Well, let me call him."

"I am not letting *you* call the sheriff at three in the morning because then we'll have to explain that I allowed it to happen. Look, this is getting out of hand. You need to make a decision on what you want to do."

The patient paced some more and cried. She then began shrieking loudly and threw one of her bags across the lobby.

"Ma'am," the officer said, "I *will* arrest you for

disorderly conduct. Now, I don't want to do that because then you become my problem for the night, but you'd do best if you keep your temper in check and make a decision about where you want to go from here. These nice women here can help you, if you want to see a doctor. If you don't, but you want to seek help for substance abuse, we can still contact that rehab facility. You're running out of time to make a choice. Pretty soon we're going to make it for you. You can't stay here and continue this all night."

"I'm going to call my husband again," she said.

The officer shook his head. "He told me not to let you call back."

The woman tried to push past the cop. The other officer drew his taser.

"Let me call him," she argued. "You can't stop me. This is a free country. I have freedom of speech, man. Read the bible."

I wanted to chuckle, but I was trying to focus in case the officer decided to tase the patient. I sure didn't want to miss that.

"Okay," the officer sighed. "I'm giving you ten seconds to make a decision. You either get your stuff and get out, see a doctor, or go to jail. Clock starts now."

The woman panicked and then asked, "Can you drop me off somewhere? I can't carry all my bags."

The officer seemed relieved. The other put his taser back on his belt.

"Where would you like me to drop you off?"

The patient gave someone's name.

"And who is that?"

"The president of the First Savings and Loan."

"I'm not taking you there. Anywhere else?"

"My daughter's house."

"And where is that?"

The patient gave a town located five hours away.

"I can't drive you five hours away," the officer stated.

The patient pouted. "But you just told me you'd give me a ride. You're a liar. All men are liars. You all like to get our hopes up, promise us great futures, promise to give us the world. But then you rip our hearts out and all your lies start coming unraveled, and you keep lying until you're standing in the living room naked."

Okay, I laughed at that one.

This caused the patient to turn to me.

Crap.

"Honey," she said to me, "you're a woman. Take me to my daughter's house. We'll have a grand time."

"Uh, no," I opted out. "I'm working and I really don't want to be in a car with you."

"We can start all over again, both of us. I bet you don't have anything here worth keeping. You work for commies, sweetie."

The police finally agreed to drive the patient to the county line, where she wanted to go, but they never got that far. As the patient was walking to the police car, she went berserk and threw one of her bags at one of the officers.

She was promptly arrested, and the whole scene ended just about two and a half hours after she originally came to the registration desk.

Thanks for the Notice

Patients often bring their doctor's orders to the Emergency Room registration desk so they can be registered for lab work. Every now and then, a patient will bring in their bodily samples and an order. I take everything from the patient, register him/her, and then call the lab so a tech can come over and pick up the samples.

Most of the time, this goes well.

Yeah, this time, it didn't.

A female patient approached the desk with a tied Wal Mart bag in her hand. She handed me the bag and I placed it on the counter next to me.

"The order is inside the bag," she told me.

And then she told me something else.

"I lost the sample cup, so I had to use a Ziploc bag."

"Uh," I replied hesitantly, "okay."

The woman left and I opened the Wal Mart bag to retrieve the order.

Now, the patient either didn't know or decided not to tell me the Wal Mart bag was leaking. And she also neglected to mention or didn't find it necessary to mention that the sample in question was diarrhea being tested for C-Diff. Now, anyone who's ever smelled C-Diff can tell you right off the bat what it is. I almost gagged.

I still had to enter the patient's information in the computer and couldn't do that without the diarrhea-stained order. I grabbed a pair of latex gloves and situated the order on top of the leaking Ziploc bag and proceeded to register the patient.

When I was finished, I wanted the entire bag as far away from me as possible, so I tied up the Wal Mart bag again and lifted it from the counter. It wasn't until I was halfway to the back office that I noticed *that* bag had a hole, too...and I had diarrhea all down the leg of my pants.

Nothing's Worse than Ballet

A husband trying to get out of going out on a date night with his wife decided to intentionally aim a nail gun at his hand and shoot. It certainly worked to get him out of the date. The six-inch-long nail went straight through the patient's thumbnail and was sticking out the other side. Due to the nail having a hooked tip, doctors had to clip the nail from either side and pull out the leftover piece. The man's wife was pissed. She left him at the hospital and told him to find his own ride home.

Real Chief Complaint from a Teenage Patient at the Registration Desk:

"I feel sick when I smoke, so I'm pretty sure I'm pregnant."

Tests confirmed she was.

Her main concern:

"Can you give me something so I can still smoke without puking?"

Daddy's Little Girl

"Nobody's going to call my dad, right?" asked a patient.

I shook my head. "You're over eighteen, so not unless you want us to."

I have to admit, I was slightly distracted by the tassels hiding her nipples.

"Good," she laughed. "He can't know where I work."

And that was at the local strip club. The patient fell off the stage during her act and sprained her ankle. She was brought to the hospital in a thong, high heel shoes, tassels hanging from her nipples, and glitter all over her skin.

In Case You Didn't Know

If you experienced flank pain *yesterday*, but you woke up *today* and felt fine, you're not really making any friends by coming to the ER and using this as your chief complaint when we have a line of people waiting to be seen trailing out the door.

Let's Just Walk Away from This

Near the end of the slowest overnight shift *ever*, a very-pregnant young woman and her husband entered the ER. The woman's husband was in a wheelchair. Both of his legs had been amputated at just below the knees. His wife declined my offer to get her a wheelchair, stating she was uncomfortable and would prefer to stand.

I registered the patient and called to the OB floor to let them know a patient 'positive' she was in labor (and she 'absolutely' knew because she had seven other kids at home) was on the way.

As I was wrapping up the registration process, the charge nurse walked through triage and stood by the copier.

"It's an OB," I said. "They're not coming through ER."

"Good," she smiled.

And then she tried to joke with the patient and her husband.

"Well, look at this," she laughed, motioning to the patient's husband. "She's the one having the baby, yet you're the one in the wheelchair."

Oh no. It was clear the nurse didn't know why.

She continued, "You should switch places. You should walk and she can relax."

The patient and her husband were quiet and I turned my head slowly to look at the nurse with the most 'I can't believe you said that' expression on my face.

"Well," she waved, "good luck, guys."

She then went back to the back, where all the nurses were singing Barry Manilow music loudly.

"Uh," I stammered to the patient's husband, "I'm so sorry about that."

He flicked his wrist. "Don't worry about it. She didn't know."

An orderly came downstairs and took the patient and her husband to the OB floor.

A few minutes later, the phone rang and I answered. It was the charge nurse.

"Okay. You looked at me strangely when those patients came in. Did the husband come in in a wheelchair?"

I bit my lip and said, "Yes. He was an amputee."

"He was an amputee?" she exclaimed.

It was apparent, by the laughter and groans of the other nurses, that she mentioned the situation to everyone in back.

"Well," she nervously chuckled, "I guess I sure put my foot in my mouth."

Once she realized that wasn't any better, she simply hung up.

You Came in for That?

Real patient complaints at the time of registration include:

* "His baby sister threw a three-pound rock at him four days ago. I just really thought I should finally get it checked out (at 02:30, when the kid had to be at school the next morning), so here we are."

* "I told the girl at the salon she had my weave too tight and said I'd sue her if she damaged my scalp. I need someone to look at my hair."

* "I may have swallowed a tack. I don't remember spitting it out."

* "My baby's poop smells."

* "I slept after I left here this morning, then got up. But then I tried to sleep again and wasn't tired. I have insomnia."

* "A dog knocked me down and now my butt hurts. And can I get a pregnancy test, too?"

* "My nose itches."

* Hiccups for four days

* Possible allergic reaction after ingesting strawberry-flavored sexual lubricant

* A patient checked in for hand pain. When I went to his room to ask more questions, he said he punched a wall because his girlfriend wanted to watch *Frozen* again, and it would make "like, the tenth time in two days."

* "My pee smells like asparagus. It's weird, too, because I ate that last night."

* Possible overdose after drinking homemade alcohol. The homemade alcohol was made with glass cleaner.

* Rock/jewelry/food stuck in ear

* Premature ejaculation

* "My dog keeps sniffing my hands and I think I may have cancer because I heard if a dog

sniffs part of your body for a long time, that means it really smells the cancer that is growing inside of you." The patient neglected to say she also prepared mixed meatloaf with her hands and didn't wash when she was finished.

* A patient explained she overate at a party and ended up consuming a plate of jalapeno poppers. She was in the ER because she later had a bowel movement that scared her. "It's never burned so bad in my life," she said.

* "I think I have [Ebola, the measles, listeria]." If it's in the news, at least two people are going to show up at the ER and be convinced they have it.

* Sunburn

* Bad breath

Just Sayin'

If you're concerned about the waiting time before you even register, or you threaten to leave because the "wait is too long," you're probably not experiencing an emergency in the first place. This department was designed for patients presenting problems that would make leaving and going home the last thing they ever did.

Order Up

A male patient came in for groin pain, testicular swelling, and burning with urination. Several doctors had been in and out of the man's room, telling him a test would be ordered for his urine. He apparently forgot this when the nurse handed him a specimen cup.

The patient went to the bathroom and was in there a lot longer than anyone expected.

He returned to his room and left his filled specimen cup on the counter.

When his nurse came in, he asked her, "Is that enough?"

The cup was filled with semen, not urine.

That HAS to be It

A middle-aged male and female approached the registration desk one evening.

"How can I help you?" I asked.

The woman seemed angry. "He needs tested."

I hesitated. "Like, STD testing or...?"

"If he needed tested for that, I would've said that," she snapped.

"So what kind of testing do you feel you need, sir?"

The wife answered, "He needs to be tested for, like, ADD or ADHD or something like that."

I asked the man his information, but he stood quietly, almost as if his wife didn't allow him to speak.

Once we registered the man, I sent him to the waiting room.

"This man is almost fifty," the triage nurse commented to me in a whisper. "What's going on here?"

I shrugged. "He hasn't talked at all. The wife answered everything. She seems pushy."

"Okay, thanks."

The triage nurse called the patient back to the triage room and invited him to sit down.

She asked the normal questions, to which the wife replied.

"And what makes you think you need testing for ADD or ADHD, *sir*?"

The patient's wife started to reply.

"Let me hear it from the patient," the nurse interrupted. "Sometimes it helps us best to hear the *patient* explain what's going on."

The patient's wife was angry. "I can tell you just as well as he can. You see, he looks at other women. All the time, he does. When we go to the mall, I catch him sneaking peeks. He watches porn on TV after I go to bed. He's always looking at other women."

"I told you," the patient finally spoke, "I can't help it. I have to look."

"See?" the wife yelled. "He needs medication because he can't focus on his marriage. He's too distracted by other women."

Emergency Room Bingo

Cold & flu symptoms	A patient with such strong B.O. you have to smear Vicks under your nose before going in the room	Toothache	"How long is the wait right now?"	ETOH
Security is paged to a patient's room	Alt LOC in otherwise healthy adult	"What's on the dinner menu tonight?"	Migraine	Stemi
Scabies	Convenient Care sent PT to ER	**FREE**	"Can I get back to see...?"	PT Unresponsive
Fight in waiting room	PT is <2 years old	Flank pain	Frequent Flyer	Vomiting
Left before triage	Multiple ambulances in bay	PT is >80 years old	Coughing	Psych Eval

One Last Thing:

Your grandmother was right. Always wear clean underwear. You never quite know when you'll end up in the ER, and once that cute doctor sees your skid marks, they can't be unseen.

Hey, readers!

If you noticed a spelling/grammatical/formatting error in this book, please feel free to review this book and let me know. You deserve the best product, and I don't always catch my mistakes (despite lots of editing and reviewing).

Thank you for your help, and thanks for reading!

A Post-Publication Message to My Readers...

If you're reading this, you must be new to the series or have decided to return to the start of this series to have a binge-reading session. Either way, thank you for your support!

I wrote this book after taking advice from friends and family. I never thought I would write another, yet the tenth edition of *Real Stories from a Small-Town ER* is on its way.

This first book is unique, as I tried to write with great detail and keep my sarcasm at bay. By the time I started the second book, that was no longer an option. These books have become fantastic stress relief tools, and readers seem to appreciate the humor and realness of the other books.

Still, I can't ignore the book that started it all!

Thank you ALL for your support.

I read every review on Amazon and would love to hear from you. You can also follow me on Twitter or Facebook.

Have a great day!

Made in the USA
Lexington, KY
20 January 2019